Study Guide
to Accompany

FUNDAMENTALS OF NURSING

FOURTH EDITION

D1515438

Study Guide to Accompany

FUNDAMENTALS OF NURSING

STANDARDS & PRACTICE

FOURTH EDITION

Sue C. DeLaune MN, RN

Assistant Professor
School of Nursing
William Carey University
New Orleans, Louisiana
President and Educational Director
SDeLaune Consulting
Mandeville, Louisiana

Patricia K. Ladner MS, MN, RN

Former Consultant for Nursing
Practice
Louisiana State Board of Nursing
New Orleans, Louisiana

prepared by

Dawna Martich, RN, MSN
Nurse Education Consultant
Pittsburgh, Pennsylvania

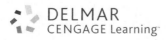
DELMAR
CENGAGE Learning™

Australia • Canada • Mexico • Singapore • Spain • United Kingdom • United States

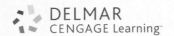
DELMAR
CENGAGE Learning™

Study Guide to Accompany Fundamentals of Nursing: Standards and Practice, Fourth Edition
Sue C. DeLaune and Patricia K. Ladner
Prepared by Dawna Martich

Vice President, Career and Professional Editorial: Dave Garza

Director of Learning Solutions: Matthew Kane

Executive Editor: Stephen Helba

Managing Editor: Marah Bellegarde

Senior Product Manager: Patricia A. Gaworecki

Editorial Assistant: Meghan Orvis

Vice President, Career and Professional Marketing: Jennifer Ann Baker

Marketing Director: Wendy E. Mapstone

Senior Marketing Manager: Michele McTighe

Marketing Coordinator: Scott A. Chrysler

Production Director: Carolyn Miller

Production Manager: Andrew Crouth

Senior Content Project Manager: Kenneth McGrath

Art Director: Jack Pendleton

© 2011, 2006, 2002, 1998 Delmar, Cengage Learning

ALL RIGHTS RESERVED. No part of this work covered by the copyright herein may be reproduced, transmitted, stored, or used in any form or by any means graphic, electronic, or mechanical, including but not limited to photocopying, recording, scanning, digitizing, taping, Web distribution, information networks, or information storage and retrieval systems, except as permitted under Section 107 or 108 of the 1976 United States Copyright Act, without the prior written permission of the publisher.

For product information and technology assistance, contact us at
Cengage Learning Customer & Sales Support, 1-800-354-9706

For permission to use material from this text or product, submit all requests online at **www.cengage.com/permissions.**
Further permissions questions can be e-mailed to
permissionrequest@cengage.com

Example: Microsoft ® is a registered trademark of the Microsoft Corporation.

Library of Congress Control Number: 2009938742

ISBN-13: 978-1-4354-8068-1
ISBN-10: 1-4354-8068-6

Delmar
5 Maxwell Drive
Clifton Park, NY 12065-2919
USA

Cengage Learning is a leading provider of customized learning solutions with office locations around the globe, including Singapore, the United Kingdom, Australia, Mexico, Brazil, and Japan. Locate your local office at: **international.cengage.com/region**

Cengage Learning products are represented in Canada by Nelson Education, Ltd.

To learn more about Delmar, visit **www.cengage.com/delmar**
Purchase any of our products at your local college store or at our preferred online store **www.CengageBrain.com**

Notice to the Reader
Publisher does not warrant or guarantee any of the products described herein or perform any independent analysis in connection with any of the product information contained herein. Publisher does not assume, and expressly disclaims, any obligation to obtain and include information other than that provided to it by the manufacturer. The reader is expressly warned to consider and adopt all safety precautions that might be indicated by the activities described herein and to avoid all potential hazards. By following the instructions contained herein, the reader willingly assumes all risks in connection with such instructions. The publisher makes no representations or warranties of any kind, including but not limited to, the warranties of fitness for particular purpose or merchantability, nor are any such representations implied with respect to the material set forth herein, and the publisher takes no responsibility with respect to such material. The publisher shall not be liable for any special, consequential, or exemplary damages resulting, in whole or part, from the readers' use of, or reliance upon, this material.

Printed in the United States of America
1 2 3 4 5 6 7 12 11 10

Table of Contents

UNIT 5: RESPONDING TO BASIC PSYCHOSOCIAL NEEDS

UNIT 6: RESPONDING TO BASIC PHYSIOLOGICAL NEEDS

Chapter 1 Evolution of Nursing and Nursing Education

1. Currently the nursing profession sees itself as focusing on

   a. illness.

   b. responses to illness for the person or community.

   c. prescribing practitioner satisfaction with the level of care.

   d. relieving the nursing shortage.

2. Prior to the use of the term *registered nurse* to identify an educated and licensed nurse, nurses were considered _____.

3. For the nursing profession to advance, nursing education must

   a. concern itself with how the profession should evolve.

   b. concern itself with its beliefs and values.

   c. respond to the changes that occur in society and health care.

   d. provide graduates with competencies to meet the health care challenges of the twenty-first century.

4. Florence Nightingale revolutionized nursing by

   a. establishing the first hospital in Britain where nurses could practice without the direction of prescribing practitioners.

   b. changing the image of nurses from handmaidens to professionals with autonomy.

   c. educating nurses in theoretical concepts as well as clinical skills.

   d. developing the first documentation system for client care.

© 2011 Cengage Learning. All Rights Reserved. May not be scanned, copied or duplicated, or posted to a publicly accessible website, in whole or in part.

5. Which of the following women in nursing history founded the Red Cross in the United States?

   a. Dorothea Dix

   b. Lillian Wald

   c. Annie Goodrich

   d. Clara Barton

6. Which of the following nursing leaders founded several nursing organizations and supported the rights of nursing students?

   a. Isabel Hampton Robb

   b. Adelaide Nutting

   c. Jane Delano

   d. Lavinia Dock

7. _____ was the first state to pass a nurse registration law.

   a. California

   b. New Mexico

   c. New York

   d. North Carolina

8. Match the decade in the left column with the event that occurred in that decade from the right column.

   _____ 1920s   a. Proliferation of HMOs

   _____ 1930s   b. Creation of Medicare and Medicaid

   _____ 1940s   c. The Brown report

   _____ 1950s   d. Women can vote

   _____ 1960s   e. The advent of Blue Cross and Blue Shield

   _____ 1970s   f. The advent of LPN programs

   _____ 1980s   g. Health care reform

   _____ 1990s   h. Nurse practitioners reimbursed directly for their services

© 2011 Cengage Learning. All Rights Reserved. May not be scanned, copied or duplicated, or posted to a publicly accessible website, in whole or in part.

9. Which of the following nursing leaders established the Frontier Nursing Service, thereby introducing health care delivery to rural America?

    a.   Mary Breckinridge

    b.   Adelaide Nutting

    c.   Clara Barton

    d.   Lavinia Dock

10. _____ was the nurse leader most known for activist work around the issue of birth control and contraception.

    a.   Adah Belle Thoms

    b.   Margaret Sanger

    c.   Jane Delano

    d.   Annie Goodrich

11. Several landmark reports about medical and nursing education brought about changes in nursing. Match the report with its focus listed in the right column.

_____	Flexner report	a.	Identified a shortage of nurses in teaching, research, and administration
_____	Goldmark report	b.	Brought accountability to medical education
_____	Brown report	c.	Identified the need for greater professional competence in nursing; recommended moving nursing education from hospitals to the university setting
_____	Nursing and Nursing Education: Public Policies and Private Actions	d.	Identified major weaknesses in hospital-based nursing programs

12. Which of the following nursing pioneers suggested the establishment of a national health insurance plan?

    a.   Isabel Hampton Robb

    b.   Lillian Wald

    c.   Adelaide Nutting

    d.   Mary Mahoney

© 2011 Cengage Learning. All Rights Reserved. May not be scanned, copied or duplicated, or posted to a publicly accessible website, in whole or in part.

13. The main reason for the growth of insurance plans in the 1920s was

    a. physician advocacy.

    b. the influence of the Metropolitan Life Insurance Company.

    c. the Depression.

    d. pressure from hospitals.

14. The proliferation of practical nursing programs in the 1950s was due to

    a. a need for nurses to work at lower wages.

    b. the cost to attend a registered nurse training program.

    c. the difficulty of being admitted to a registered nurse educational program.

    d. the need to increase the supply of nurses.

15. During the Civil War, nurses who provided care to the ill and injured were

    a. sisters of religious orders.

    b. male nurse-priests.

    c. volunteers.

    d. wives and female relatives of the soldiers.

16. The organization that guides staff development activities is the

    a. American Nurses Association.

    b. state board of nursing.

    c. National League for Nursing.

    d. Joint Commission.

17. The Healthy People initiatives are considered the nation's health agenda. What is the purpose of this agenda?

    a. To reduce health care costs

    b. To increase the number of practicing nurses in the United States

    c. To promote healthful activities and prevent disease

    d. To ensure adequate funding for Medicare and Medicaid

© 2011 Cengage Learning. All Rights Reserved. May not be scanned, copied or duplicated, or posted to a publicly accessible website, in whole or in part.

18. According to differentiated nursing practice, the BSN-prepared nurse would provide care in

   a. nursing homes.

   b. hospitals with care management and the community.

   c. independent practices and as a primary provider.

   d. extended care and assisted living facilities.

19. What must exist in a profession in order to achieve autonomy?

   a. Empowerment

   b. Satisfaction

   c. Commitment

   d. Quality education

20. Which of the following is an innovative approach to meet the need for 1 million additional nurses by the year 2010?

   a. Increased salary for nurses

   b. Reduced overtime hours

   c. Differentiated practice

   d. Accelerated degree programs

Critical Thinking

21. What concepts of nursing did Nightingale introduce that are still being utilized in nursing today?

22. Discuss why nursing education today includes preparation for natural disasters, highly communicable diseases, and terrorist attacks.

© 2011 Cengage Learning. All Rights Reserved. May not be scanned, copied or duplicated, or posted to a publicly accessible website, in whole or in part.

Activities

23. Break into small groups and discuss the advantages and disadvantages of having different levels of entry into the profession of nursing.

24. Invite a panel of advanced practice nurses to the class to discuss the following:

    a. Their roles

    b. Why they chose to advance their practice

    c. What challenges they face as advanced practice nurses

    d. What they do differently now that they are advanced practice nurses

25. Invite a variety of nurse educators to the class. Discuss the similarities and differences between a clinical instructor, a college/university professor, a staff development instructor/trainer, and a disease-specific (diabetes, enterostomal) nurse educator.

26. Access the National Council for the State Boards of Nursing Web site and research continuing education requirements for different states. Discuss which states have mandatory course requirements and which do not.

© 2011 Cengage Learning. All Rights Reserved. May not be scanned, copied or duplicated, or posted to a publicly accessible website, in whole or in part.

Chapter 2   Nursing Theory

1. Match the definitions from the right column with the terms in the left column.

    _____ concept   a. The use of formalized methods to generate information about a phenomenon

    _____ phenomenon   b. A relational statement that links concepts

    _____ proposition   c. Basic building block of theory

    _____ theory   d. Field of study

    _____ discipline   e. An observable fact that can be perceived through the senses and explained

    _____ research   f. Describes, explains, or predicts situations

2. Nursing practice, theory, and research exist

    a. independently of each other.

    b. as a closely related whole.

    c. in a loosely linked relationship.

    d. to validate interventions.

3. Which of the following would represent a grand nursing theory?

    a. Peplau's theory of interpersonal relations

    b. Orem's self-care deficit theory of nursing

    c. Nightingale's *Notes on Nursing*

    d. Abdellah's 21 nursing problems

4. Nursing theory development and research activities are directed toward

    _____.

© 2011 Cengage Learning. All Rights Reserved. May not be scanned, copied or duplicated, or posted to a publicly accessible website, in whole or in part.

5. The unifying force in a discipline that names the phenomena of concern to that discipline is called a

   a. paradigm.

   b. metaparadigm.

   c. framework.

   d. model.

6. The exploration of a nursing theory provides the nurse with

   a. new insights into client care.

   b. expanded beliefs about nursing care.

   c. stronger nursing role models.

   d. a mechanism for the nurse to think about nursing.

7. According to Fawcett, the major concepts that provide structure to the domain of nursing are

   a. client, environment, health, nursing.

   b. nursing, client, environment, health.

   c. person, environment, nursing, well-being.

   d. person, environment, health, nursing.

8. The theorists who view the discipline of nursing as fitting the "totality paradigm" are all of the following except

   a. Imogene King.

   b. Dorothea Orem.

   c. Jean Watson.

   d. Sr. Callista Roy.

9. Which nursing theorist put forward the following definition of nursing? "The unique function of the nurse is to assist the individual, sick or well, in the performance of those activities contributing to health or its recovery (or to peaceful death) that he would perform unaided if he had the necessary strength, will, or knowledge."

   a. Florence Nightingale

   b. Jean Watson

   c. Myra Levine

   d. Virginia Henderson

© 2011 Cengage Learning. All Rights Reserved. May not be scanned, copied or duplicated, or posted to a publicly accessible website, in whole or in part.

10. A client recovering from surgery experiences a stroke and needs to learn how to swallow. The nurse supports the adaptive behavior to maximize functioning. Which theory best describes the care needed to support the client's coping?

    a.   Orem's self-care deficit theory of nursing

    b.   The Roy adaptation model

    c.   Watson's human caring theory

    d.   King's goal attainment theory

11. How does nursing practice support nursing theory?

    a.   It provides the raw material for the ideas that are organized in the form of nursing theory.

    b.   It validates ideas.

    c.   It is used to transform nursing theory.

    d.   It influences the development of nursing theory.

12. Which of the following nursing theorists is concerned with a humanistic-altruistic philosophical basis for the science of nursing as well as the classification of caring behaviors?

    a.   Jean Watson

    b.   Martha Rogers

    c.   Rosemarie Parse

    d.   Dorothea Orem

13. A middle-range theory provides a perspective from which to view complex situations and a direction for nursing interventions. Which theorist proposed a middle-range theory?

    a.   Maslow

    b.   Erikson

    c.   Selye

    d.   Peplau

© 2011 Cengage Learning. All Rights Reserved. May not be scanned, copied or duplicated, or posted to a publicly accessible website, in whole or in part.

14. In a conversation with two nurse colleagues, you hear a discussion about the scope of practice of the various helping disciplines. When discussing the difference between medicine and nursing, Nurse A says medicine and nursing share the same metaparadigm, citing that nurses carry out prescribing practitioners' orders. Nurse B states that the metaparadigm of nursing is broader than that of medicine. Which of these nurses represents the perspective aligned with current nursing theory and practice?

    a. Nurse A

    b. Nurse B

    c. Neither

    d. Both

15. The concept of homeostasis becomes obsolete when considering the theory of which of the following theorists?

    a. Jean Watson

    b. Dorothea Orem

    c. Martha Rogers

    d. Sr. Callista Roy

16. Nursing theory development began with the writings of Florence Nightingale in 1859. Place the following nursing theories in sequence from earliest development to most recent.

    _____ Jean Watson: *The philosophy and science of caring*

    _____ Martha Rogers: *A Science of Unitary Man*

    _____ Virginia Henderson: *The Nature of Nursing*

    _____ Dorothea Orem: self-care deficit theory of nursing

    _____ Rosemarie Parse: *Man-Living-Health: A Theory of Nursing*

    _____ Myra Levine: the four conservation principles

    _____ Patricia Benner: *From Novice to Expert*

    _____ Madeline Leininger: *Culture Care Diversity and Universality*

    _____ Faye Abdellah: 21 nursing problems

17. Existentialism influenced the work of this early nursing theorist who focused her work on the human-to-human relationship and the meaning in experiences such as illness. Who was this theorist?

    a. Joyce Travelbee

    b. Faye Abdellah

    c. Myra Levine

    d. Patricia Benner

© 2011 Cengage Learning. All Rights Reserved. May not be scanned, copied or duplicated, or posted to a publicly accessible website, in whole or in part.

18. Which of the following nursing theories is consistent with the simultaneity paradigm?

  a. Martha Rogers

  b. Myra Levine

  c. Dorothea Orem

  d. Sr. Callista Roy

19. Mr. Hill, 38 years old, is a newly diagnosed diabetic. Since he is to be discharged tomorrow, you are reviewing aspects of his self-care regimen. You teach, reinforce, and ask for a demonstration of his ability to self-administer insulin injections. At the completion of the teaching session, he asks you to return later to review how to draw up insulin in a syringe. Which of the following theories would best describe the theoretical framework you will be operating through as you meet his self-care need?

  a. Orem's theory

  b. Watson's theory

  c. Levigne's theory

20. Emphasis in nursing theory has changed from developing new theories to including additional concepts such as

  a. cultural diversity and family.

  b. weight management and diabetes control.

  c. smoking cessation and exercise.

  d. recreational activities and the meaning of life.

Critical Thinking

21. Explain how prevention and wellness represent a paradigm shift within the health care industry.

22. What are "real life" examples of the simultaneity paradigm?

Activities

23. At your current level of nursing education, identify the nursing theorist who best exemplifies your current experience with the nursing profession. Explain why you chose that theorist.

24. Using the Internet, research the disciplines of sociology and behavioral health to identify other nonnursing theories that nursing utilizes for the provision of client care.

© 2011 Cengage Learning. All Rights Reserved. May not be scanned, copied or duplicated, or posted to a publicly accessible website, in whole or in part.

Chapter 3   Research and Evidence-Based Practice

1. Exploratory research is defined as

   a. research studies in which the investigator controls the independent variable and randomly assigns subjects to different conclusions.

   b. investigations that have as their main objective the accurate portrayal of characteristics of persons, groups, or situations.

   c. studies in which the subjects cannot be randomly assigned to treatment conditions.

   d. preliminary investigation designed to develop or refine a hypothesis or to test data collection methods.

2. The first doctoral degree program for nurses was offered by

   a. New York University in 1915.

   b. University of Indiana in 1933.

   c. Columbus University in 1923.

   d. Yale University in 1929.

3. An example of instrumental research utilization is

   a. adopting a new dressing change protocol that improves wound healing.

   b. petitioning the nursing director for more staff.

   c. suggesting alternative solutions to a nurse-client ratio issue.

   d. meeting with government officials to change state smoking laws.

4. In today's health care environment, the challenge to nurses is to determine the interrelatedness of nursing research to

   a. medication management.

   b. care planning.

   c. creation of critical pathways.

   d. evidence-based practice.

© 2011 Cengage Learning. All Rights Reserved. May not be scanned, copied or duplicated, or posted to a publicly accessible website, in whole or in part.

5. The Western Interstate Commission for Higher Education's Regional Program for Nursing Research Development was the first federally funded research project. Which component did it include?

    a. Identification of research studies and establishment of a research base

    b. Transformation of findings into research-based protocols

    c. Evaluation of the effects of change

    d. Evaluation of research-based practice

6. In nursing research, the primary source is defined as

    a. an article written by one or more researchers.

    b. revised research.

    c. research cited in a text or paper.

    d. the first time a source is cited.

7. The four parts of an evidence report are

    a. statement, evidence, analysis, and best practice.

    b. statement, analysis, evidence, and recommendations.

    c. analysis, evidence, synthesis, and recommendations.

    d. evidence, hypothesis, best practice, and recommendations.

8. Which statement best describes evidence-based practice?

    a. It is a best practice.

    b. It is the easiest intervention.

    c. It is the safest intervention.

    d. It is the best evidence available to guide clinical decision making.

9. What are the three elements required in the integrated approach to the daily practice of nursing?

    a. Best practice guidelines, full disclosure, and research

    b. Research, practice, and analysis

    c. Research, education, and practice

    d. Education, practice, and analysis

© 2011 Cengage Learning. All Rights Reserved. May not be scanned, copied or duplicated, or posted to a publicly accessible website, in whole or in part.

10. Nursing has historically acquired knowledge through a variety of methods. One method is basing practice on customs and past trends. This is considered

    a. tradition.

    b. authority.

    c. borrowing.

    d. trial and error.

11. Which of the following would likely lead to the implementation of evidence-based nursing practice?

    a. Efforts to change the behavior of the individual nurse

    b. The design of organizational systems that facilitate change

12. Which type of research involves the systematic collection of numerical data, often under considerable control?

    a. Quantitative

    b. Qualitative

    c. Historical

    d. Summative

13. Match the term in the left column with its definition from the right column.

    _____ hypothesis   a. Variation of a variable

    _____ independent variable b. Statement of relationship between two variables

    _____ dependent variable   c. Abstraction inferred from situations or behaviors

    _____ construct   d. Outcome variable of interest

    _____ value   e. Controlled variable

14. When conducting a research study, the researcher informs the participants that all information collected will be kept confidential. Which human right does this define?

    a. Fair treatment

    b. Informed consent

    c. Anonymity

    d. Privacy

© 2011 Cengage Learning. All Rights Reserved. May not be scanned, copied or duplicated, or posted to a publicly accessible website, in whole or in part.

15. Which of the following statements most accurately describes the role of the nurse without a graduate degree in the research process?

   a. Designs research projects

   b. Integrates research findings into care protocol changes

   c. Collects research data as part of a research team

   d. Acts as the principal investigator on a project

16. The following are all barriers to utilizing nursing research except

   a. inadequate research.

   b. resistance to change.

   c. resource constraint.

   d. an institutional nursing research program designed to implement and generate current practice guidelines.

17. The nurse researcher is preparing the abstract for a research article. Which element will be included in the methodology section of the abstract?

   a. Problem statement

   b. Findings

   c. Sample size

   d. Framework used

18. A nurse is researching on the Internet for information about clinical practice guidelines designed to improve the quality of care and reduce costs. Which site would be most beneficial to consult?

   a. *www.jcaho.org*

   b. *www.nlnac.org*

   c. *www.aacn.nche.edu*

   d. *www.ahrq.gov/clinic/epc*

19. Evidence-based nursing practice is

   a. nursing research.

   b. the best nursing practice standard available to guide clinical decisions.

   c. a scientific rationale for nursing.

   d. an observation about best nursing care.

© 2011 Cengage Learning. All Rights Reserved. May not be scanned, copied or duplicated, or posted to a publicly accessible website, in whole or in part.

20. Research utilization occurs at which three levels?

    a. Symbiotic, conceptual, and incidental

    b. Symbolic, conceptual, and incidental

    c. Conceptual, instrumental, and symbolic

    d. Symbiotic, conceptual, and instrumental

Critical Thinking

21. A nurse is asked to participate in a research study to measure the speed in which a specific medication causes a spontaneous abortion, and the nurse does not support abortion. What should the nurse do?

22. Explain the difference between best practice and evidence-based practice.

Activities

23. Divide the class into evenly distributed groups, and have each group determine a client care problem that could serve as the topic of a research study. Once the problem is identified, work through the entire research process, including

    a. definition of the purpose.

    b. literature review.

    c. development of a conceptual framework.

    d. development of research objectives, questions, and hypotheses.

    e. definition of variables.

    f. selection of a research design.

    g. definition of the population, sample, and setting.

24. Access the Web site for the National Guideline Clearinghouse at http://www.guideline.gov. Research how to

    a. submit guidelines for consideration.

    b. locate one guideline "in progress."

    c. find client resources.

    d. find recent U.S. Food and Drug Administration advisories.

© 2011 Cengage Learning. All Rights Reserved. May not be scanned, copied or duplicated, or posted to a publicly accessible website, in whole or in part.

Chapter 4   Health Care Delivery, Quality, and the Continuum of Care

1. A client is admitted to a rehabilitation facility to recover from surgery for a hip fracture. This facility is considered

    a. primary.

    b. secondary.

    c. tertiary.

    d. palliative.

2. A prescribing practitioner who is reimbursed directly by an insurance company for services provided is being reimbursed by which method?

    a. Capitation

    b. Fee-for-service

    c. Single-payer method

    d. Managed care

3. State the three issues health care reform must address.

    a. _____

    b. _____

    c. _____

4. Match the managed care model in the left column with its appropriate characteristic from the right column.

    _____ HMO (health maintenance organization)

    _____ PPO (preferred provider organization)

    _____ EPO (exclusive provider organization)

    a. Care must be delivered by the plan in order for clients to receive reimbursement.

    b. Focus on care is on cost-effective treatment measures with quality outcomes.

    c. Members are limited to providers within the system.

© 2011 Cengage Learning. All Rights Reserved. May not be scanned, copied or duplicated, or posted to a publicly accessible website, in whole or in part.

5. Match the term with the correct definition.

   _____ quality assurance

   _____ continuous quality improvement

   _____ total quality management

   a. Approach to quality management in which scientific approaches are used to study work processes

   b. Method of management and system operation used to achieve continuous improvement

   c. Traditional approach to quality management in which individual performance is evaluated

6. List the three federal programs for reimbursing health care.

   a. _____

   b. _____

   c. _____

7. Which of the following is one reason why a nursing shortage is imminent?

   a. Pharmaceutical industry cutbacks

   b. Restructuring health care

   c. Location of health care facilities

   d. Declining number of nursing faculty

8. Which group spurred the movement toward cost containment of health care?

   a. Prescribing practitioners

   b. Insurance companies

   c. The business sector

   d. The American Association of Retired Persons (AARP)

9. The major purposes of health care are to promote _____ and prevent _____ or _____.

10. Which health care service is provided through primary care?

    a. Diagnosis

    b. Teaching

    c. Surgery

© 2011 Cengage Learning. All Rights Reserved. May not be scanned, copied or duplicated, or posted to a publicly accessible website, in whole or in part.

11.   Which agency is responsible for administering the Medicare and Medicaid programs?

   a.   CMS

   b.   Joint Commission

   c.   American Nurses Association

   d.   National League for Nurses

12.   If a health care organization fails to adhere to quality standards for care, which of the following can occur?

   a.   Duplication of work between departments

   b.   New staff recruitment and retraining

   c.   Overutilization of diagnostic tests

   d.   Denial of payment for services

13.   Which factor places the quality of hospital care at risk when hospitals restructure?

   a.   Replacing brand name medications with generic drugs

   b.   Replacing RNs with UAPs

   c.   Shortening the length of stay (LOS) for certain medical diagnoses

   d.   Blending the roles of hospital workers into a multiskilled worker

14.   One dimension of an organization's culture is atmosphere. Which characteristic is an example of the atmosphere in a high-performing organization?

   a.   Open and nonthreatening

   b.   Intimidating

   c.   Guarded

   d.   Political

15.   What is the percentage goal recommended by Healthy People 2010 for preschool children in this country to be immunized?

   a.   10%

   b.   25%

   c.   35%

   d.   40%

© 2011 Cengage Learning. All Rights Reserved. May not be scanned, copied or duplicated, or posted to a publicly accessible website, in whole or in part.

16. In *Nursing's Agenda for Health Care Reform*, a cornerstone of this proposal is that

    a. all citizens must have access to health care services.

    b. health care services should be paid for by a single payer from public funds.

    c. health care must emphasize illness cure.

    d. integrated health systems must improve the continuity of care.

17. What statement would be accurate about nurse practitioner versus prescribing practitioner care?

    a. Nurse practitioners charge more for services.

    b. Nurse practitioners spend more time with their clients.

    c. Nurse practitioners can independently diagnose and treat common acute illnesses and injures.

    d. Nurse practitioners have prescriptive privileges in all states.

18. Which action is the nurse manager's responsibility in quality improvement?

    a. Be self-directed

    b. Serve as a change agent

    c. Support colleagues

    d. Lead by example

19. A client has had a total hip replacement and is transferred to a facility for restorative care. This facility would be

    a. Hospice.

    b. a managed care organization.

    c. a community nursing center.

    d. a long-term extended-care facility.

20. According to the Centers for Medicare and Medicaid Services, "never events" will not be reimbursed with payment to hospitals. Which occurrence is an example of a never event?

    a. The wrong dose of medication is administered to a client.

    b. A client is kept on a clear liquid diet 1 day longer than necessary.

    c. A client falls out of bed and breaks her wrist.

    d. A client pulls out his indwelling urinary catheter.

© 2011 Cengage Learning. All Rights Reserved. May not be scanned, copied or duplicated, or posted to a publicly accessible website, in whole or in part.

Critical Thinking

21.   Explain why customer satisfaction is an important health care organizational goal today.

22.   Explain what is causing the cost of health care to increase.

Activities

23.   During a clinical experience, observe health care providers working with clients. Search for episodes or examples in which a health care provider offers positive customer service. Identify episodes when customer service can be improved. Be prepared to discuss these observations at the conclusion of the clinical experience.

24.   Invite CRNPs (certified registered nurse practitioners) to the class to discuss their roles in today's health care environment. Where do they work? What do they do? What are their challenges? What are their rewards?

25.   Identify a list of possible topics for which to conduct a quality improvement initiative in the clinical area. For each topic identified, determine the purpose for the initiative and the goal for improvement.

© 2011 Cengage Learning. All Rights Reserved. May not be scanned, copied or duplicated, or posted to a publicly accessible website, in whole or in part.

Chapter 5   Critical Thinking, Decision Making, and the Nursing Process

1. Match the component of critical thinking on the left with its definition on the right.

   _____ Mental operations   a. The component of critical thinking that allows a person to question assumptions

   _____ Knowledge   b. The component of critical thinking that includes decision making

   _____ Attitudes   c. The component of critical thinking that requires facts or information

2. Thorough documentation in the clinical record showing the client's responses to the nursing interventions performed is an example of _____ in action.

3. Critical thinking requires the use of a broad knowledge base to make sound clinical decisions. Which type of knowledge uses anatomical and physiological facts to solve a clinical problem?

   a. Declarative

   b. Operative

   c. Analytic

   d. Subjective

4. Which attitude is found within a critical thinker?

   a. Rigid

   b. Inflexible

   c. Closed minded

   d. Curious

© 2011 Cengage Learning. All Rights Reserved. May not be scanned, copied or duplicated, or posted to a publicly accessible website, in whole or in part.

5. Novice nurses develop clinical judgment as the length of time in nursing practice increases. Based on your understanding of critical thinking, which statement is true about the development of clinical judgment?

   a. Clinical judgment develops at the same pace for every new nurse.

   b. New knowledge is unnecessary for clinical judgment to evolve.

   c. Exploration of alternative solutions to client problems is not expected.

   d. An attitude of intellectual humility is the basis for questioning assumptions.

6. Several barriers to creative thinking have been identified in the literature. These include blocks such as being comfortable with the status quo, following tradition, operating with a rigid mindset, and going along with the majority opinion (groupthink). List two additional blocks that can interfere with creative thinking.

   a. _____

   b. _____

7. The goals of nursing outcome classification research are

   a. _____.

   b. _____.

   c. _____.

8. Match the type of nursing diagnosis from the left column with its definition from the right column.

   _____ actual diagnosis   a. Describes a potential client problem

   _____ risk diagnosis   b. Signals a situation where a problem could exist if no action is taken

   _____ possible diagnosis   c. Identifies an existing client problem

   _____ wellness diagnosis   d. Reflects a situation in which a nurse manages the client's health status with a prescribing practitioner

   _____ collaborative diagnosis   e. Reflects a desire of the client to improve health

9. Write in the type of assessment data, either *subjective* data or *objective* data.

   _____ "My head hurts."

   _____ Wound circular, 1½ inches in diameter, redness around edges, no drainage present.

   _____ "I hear voices telling me to hurt myself."

   _____ Unsteady gait, walked from bed to doorway of room.

   _____ "I am feeling upset now, I can't concentrate."

   _____ Oxygen saturation 93% on room air.

© 2011 Cengage Learning. All Rights Reserved. May not be scanned, copied or duplicated, or posted to a publicly accessible website, in whole or in part.

10. The nursing diagnosis *Impaired skin integrity* related to immobility as manifested by stage 1 pressure ulcer on coccyx is an example of which nursing diagnosis?

    a. Risk diagnosis

    b. Possible diagnosis

    c. Wellness diagnosis

    d. Actual diagnosis

11. A client is diagnosed with pneumonia. The nurse assesses the client and writes the nursing diagnosis "*Ineffective airway clearance* related to fatigue and weakness as manifested by inability to effectively cough and mobilize secretions." Which statement explains the difference between a medical and a nursing diagnosis?

    a. The nursing diagnosis is determined by the medical diagnosis.

    b. The medical diagnosis is treated by the nurse.

    c. The nursing diagnosis reflects a human response to an actual problem.

    d. Only prescribing practitioners can treat a pathophysiology.

12. Which stage of cognitive development includes the ability to form opinions and values based on weighing information in situations?

    a. Dualism

    b. Multiplicity

    c. Relativism

    d. Commitment

13. The nurse asks, "Are there any risk factors here that could affect the health of my client?" Which phase of the nursing process is the nurse using?

    a. Assessment

    b. Diagnosis

    c. Implementation

    d. Evaluation

14. An example of a priority nursing diagnosis is

    a. *Ineffective individual coping.*

    b. *Risk for injury.*

    c. *Risk for impaired skin integrity.*

    d. *Sleep pattern disturbance.*

© 2011 Cengage Learning. All Rights Reserved. May not be scanned, copied or duplicated, or posted to a publicly accessible website, in whole or in part.

15. Expected outcome statements must be realistic, have a time limit, and be

   a. clear.

   b. broad.

   c. measurable.

   d. focused.

16. A client is unable to participate in goal development. What should the nurse do?

   a. Ask the prescribing practitioner to determine the client's goals.

   b. Have the nurse manager determine the client's goals.

   c. Determine the client's goals with the input of the health care team.

   d. Determine the client's goals until the client is able to participate.

17. Which activity does the implementation phase of the nursing process include?

   a. Giving care

   b. Recording client responses

   c. Reporting significant changes

   d. All of the above

18. The nurse determines that a client's goals have been partially met. What should the nurse do?

   a. Reassess the situation.

   b. Change the time frame for completion.

   c. Change the nursing diagnosis.

   d. Start over.

© 2011 Cengage Learning. All Rights Reserved. May not be scanned, copied or duplicated, or posted to a publicly accessible website, in whole or in part.

19. In which aspect of the nursing process would a nurse use the critical thinking skill of differentiating between essential and trivial data to come to a thoughtful conclusion about a set of client signs and symptoms?

    a. Assessment

    b. Diagnosis

    c. Outcome identification

    d. Implementation

20. The nurse has completed the assessment of a client. What should the nurse do next?

    a. Plan care.

    b. Determine outcomes.

    c. Analyze the data.

    d. Choose interventions.

Critical Thinking

21. Discuss how groupthink interferes with the critical thinking process.

22. Explain the difference between a "risk" nursing diagnosis and a "possible" nursing diagnosis.

Activities

23. Identify a situation in which you had to make a decision. List the steps that you used to make the decision. Analyze each step, and show how the step relates to the critical thinking process. Discuss the decision and process used with others in the class.

24. In the clinical area, study client care plans for lists of identified nursing diagnoses. From the lists, determine which diagnoses are given priority. How many diagnoses are "actual" problems? How many diagnoses are "risks" or "possible" problems? From the lists of nursing diagnoses, determine which types of problems are identified the least often. Brainstorm reasons why some problems occur least often compared to those that are identified the most.

25. A client cannot remember to take his medication when at home. Using the critical thinking process, create a method that will facilitate the client to take his medication without fail.

© 2011 Cengage Learning. All Rights Reserved. May not be scanned, copied or duplicated, or posted to a publicly accessible website, in whole or in part.

Chapter 6   Assessment

1. A client arrives at the emergency department with the complaint of substernal chest pain. What type of assessment should be done for this client?

   a. General

   b. Comprehensive

   c. Focused

   d. Ongoing

2. Which aspect of a health history would a client most likely be reluctant to share with a nurse?

   a. Allergies

   b. Use of herbal preparations

   c. Previous hospitalizations

   d. Prescription medications

3. During the interview, a client tells the nurse that he has right ear pain. Which assessment technique would be used to best gather objective data?

   a. Palpation

   b. Inspection

   c. Percussion

   d. Auscultation

4. A client with coronary artery disease is complaining of chest pain. What should the nurse do first to help this client?

   a. Assess the location, duration, and character of the pain.

   b. Administer sublingual nitroglycerin as prescribed.

   c. Remind the client that the pain is because of a cardiac catheterization from 2 days ago.

   d. Assess the client's cardiac history.

© 2011 Cengage Learning. All Rights Reserved. May not be scanned, copied or duplicated, or posted to a publicly accessible website, in whole or in part.

5. Match the best assessment technique from the right column for determining the assessment finding in the left column.

_____	abdominal distention	a. Auscultation
_____	adventitious breath sounds	b. Palpation
_____	circumoral pallor	c. Percussion
_____	lung tissue consolidation	d. Observation

6. List four methods the nurse uses to collect data.

   a. _____

   b. _____

   c. _____

   d. _____

7. A client's heart rhythm has changed from normal sinus to atrial fibrillation, and the nurse takes a sphygmomanometer into the client's room. What information should the nurse review before assessing the client?

   a. The most recent EKG result

   b. The most recent CPK result

   c. A review of past physical illnesses

   d. The baseline vital signs

8. List the three phases of the interview process.

   a. _____

   b. _____

   c. _____

9. The best source of data about the client is the

   a. family.

   b. client's records.

   c. prescribing practitioner.

   d. client.

© 2011 Cengage Learning. All Rights Reserved. May not be scanned, copied or duplicated, or posted to a publicly accessible website, in whole or in part.

10.   A client has an oral temperature of 100°F and the complaint of burning during and frequency of urination. The nurse suspects the client has a urinary tract infection after assessing which of the following?

a.   Elevated white blood cell count

b.   Client statement about drinking large volumes of fluid

c.   Elevated bacterial cell count of the urine

d.   Client statement about the inability to wait to void

11.   In what sequence would you expect to gather information about your hospitalized clients when you first begin your work shift?

_____   The medical record, the most recent lab work results

_____   The client

_____   The care Kardex, care plan, assessment flow sheets

_____   The nurses' shift report about the client

_____   The client's family

_____   Health care personnel

12.   Match the objective and subjective data types with the following:

_____   Complaints of dizziness   a. Objective

_____   Vomiting   b. Subjective

_____   Eats only 5% of every meal

_____   States he is anxious

_____   Dressing is dry and intact

13.   A client who will be discharged in 4 days needs assistance with activities of daily living and will need to have biweekly blood work drawn once at home. What should the nurse ask the client to aid in planning his discharge needs?

a.   What assistance will you need to go to the laboratory for your blood tests?

b.   Will you need help at home?

c.   Will a family member help you at home?

d.   Do you have assistive devices at home to help you?

© 2011 Cengage Learning. All Rights Reserved. May not be scanned, copied or duplicated, or posted to a publicly accessible website, in whole or in part.

14.   A client is recovering from surgery to remove her gallbladder. She has an intravenous infusion, oxygen, a nasogastric tube set to suction, and an indwelling urinary catheter; is complaining of nausea; and received medication for pain 1 hour ago. What should the nurse assess when entering this client's room?

   a.   The position of the side rails

   b.   Wound drainage amount

   c.   Oxygen set at prescribed flow rate

   d.   Temperature of the room

15.   The purpose of the physical examination is to

   a.   determine nursing diagnoses.

   b.   plan care.

   c.   validate data obtained from the interview.

   d.   find information that the client neglected to inform caregivers about during the interview.

16.   Which of the following is of the highest importance when conducting a health history?

   a.   Food preferences

   b.   Current employer

   c.   Allergies

   d.   Recreational activities

17.   A client, prescribed digoxin, is being discharged. What should the nurse assess to help plan for the client's discharge needs?

   a.   What should you do if your pulse is below 50 beats per minute?

   b.   Where does this drug act on your body?

   c.   What are the side effects of this medication?

   d.   What pharmacy will you use to have the prescription filled?

18.   A client is admitted for surgery the next day. The nurse is planning to conduct the interview; however, the roommate has visitors and the television is loud. What should the nurse do?

   a.   Do the interview after the visitors leave the room.

   b.   Let the nurse on the next shift complete the interview.

   c.   Do the interview the morning of the surgery.

   d.   Close the curtain and ask if the television volume can be lowered.

© 2011 Cengage Learning. All Rights Reserved. May not be scanned, copied or duplicated, or posted to a publicly accessible website, in whole or in part.

19. Which of the following is done during the introduction phase of the health interview?

    a. Establish goals for the interview.

    b. Collect data.

    c. Determine the reason for seeking health care.

    d. Validate client perceptions.

20. Which assessment format is designed to document assessment data obtained from residents of a long-term care facility?

    a. The sickness impact profile

    b. The body systems model

    c. The minimum data set

    d. Maslow's hierarchy of needs

Critical Thinking

21. Discuss why the body systems model for data collection does not support the creation of nursing diagnoses.

22. A client is admitted with severe pain and is taken immediately for emergency abdominal surgery. The health history and assessment cannot be done with the client. Discuss what the nurse can do to gather information in the absence of the client's involvement.

Activities

23. Using the information provided in the list containing elements of the health history on page 94 of the textbook, pair into groups of two and practice the interview process.

24. Provide a variety of different assessment forms. (These can be obtained from different clinical sites or by searching the Internet.) For each form, determine which type of format or assessment model is used. Does the form follow a nursing model? If so, which one? If the format does not follow a nursing model, which format is used? As a group, discuss the advantages and disadvantages of using each of the different formats.

25. In the clinical area, observe a nurse conducting a client assessment. Observe for the following:

    a. Model used

    b. Techniques of assessment used and for which body area

    c. Questions or type of communication the nurse used while conducting the assessment

    d. Client responses to the assessment

© 2011 Cengage Learning. All Rights Reserved. May not be scanned, copied or duplicated, or posted to a publicly accessible website, in whole or in part.

Chapter 7   Nursing Diagnosis

1. There are similarities and differences between medical and nursing diagnoses. Which is unique to the process of establishing a nursing diagnosis?

   a. The focus is on human responses to health problems.

   b. The diagnostic process is creative and organized.

   c. Assessment data are only collected and analyzed prior to the establishment of the diagnosis.

   d. It is legally sanctioned for the profession.

2. Nursing informatics is

   a. a method of dealing with information within nursing practice.

   b. a research program.

   c. a credentialing mechanism for nurses.

   d. a specialty group in nursing.

3. The client populations identified by NANDA in *Nursing Diagnoses* (2007) that nursing diagnoses target include

   a. the individual.

   b. the family.

   c. the community.

   d. groups.

   e. all of the above.

4. The nurse reviews the nursing diagnosis definition and the defining characteristics primarily to

   a. ensure an accurate diagnosis.

   b. correlate with the medical diagnosis.

   c. validate the subjective complaints.

   d. identify a "risk for" nursing diagnosis.

© 2011 Cengage Learning. All Rights Reserved. May not be scanned, copied or duplicated, or posted to a publicly accessible website, in whole or in part.

5. The first nursing diagnosis conference in 1973 began to identify, develop, and place nursing diagnoses in a taxonomy. Which statement is correct about the nursing diagnosis taxonomy?

    a. It is a list of nursing diagnoses.

    b. It is a classification of human responses.

    c. It is a complete list of all possible diagnoses.

    d. Each nursing diagnosis has been validated using medical diagnoses as a standard.

6. Consider the nursing diagnosis *Ineffective airway clearance* R/T fatigue as evidenced by dyspnea at rest. Which portion represents the etiology for this diagnosis?

    a. Ineffective airway clearance

    b. Fatigue

    c. Dyspnea at rest

7. List a syndrome diagnosis accepted by NANDA. _____

    _____

8. The etiological component of a nursing diagnostic statement gives the cause of the problem and is written as

    a. defining characteristics.

    b. the gathered data.

    c. the "related to" factors.

    d. the objective data.

9. Which type of nursing diagnosis identifies the individual or aggregate condition or state that may be enhanced by health-promoting activities?

    a. Actual

    b. Risk

    c. Wellness

    d. Syndrome

© 2011 Cengage Learning. All Rights Reserved. May not be scanned, copied or duplicated, or posted to a publicly accessible website, in whole or in part.

10. List in sequence the steps in developing a nursing diagnosis.

_____   Data are clustered.

_____   The first part of the diagnosis is written (diagnostic label).

_____   Data cues are interpreted and assigned meaning.

_____   Related to (R/T) factors are identified and attached to the diagnosis.

_____   Data cues are identified from client data.

_____   Data cues are validated.

_____   A list of nursing diagnoses is consulted.

11. Consider the nursing diagnosis *Acute pain* R/T pain from incision. Which statement identifies the error in this nursing diagnosis?

   a.   It is saying the same thing twice.

   b.   It is using a medical diagnosis in the nursing diagnosis.

   c.   It is a judgmental statement.

   d.   It should have been written as a one-part nursing diagnosis.

12. Which would be an appropriate nursing diagnosis for an adult who is dyspneic upon exertion, has an O_2 saturation of 88%, and has crackles in both lung bases? Vital signs are BP 106/70, P 98, R 32 (at rest), T 101.2°F.

   a.   *Risk for respiratory dysfunction*

   b.   *Risk for ineffective airway clearance*

   c.   *Impaired gas exchange*

   d.   *Impaired airway clearance*

13. Which wellness nursing diagnosis is written correctly?

   a.   *Readiness for enhanced spiritual well-being*

   b.   *Enhanced spiritual well-being*

   c.   *Readiness for spiritual well-being*

   d.   *Readiness for enhanced spiritual well-being* R/T religion-seeking behavior

© 2011 Cengage Learning. All Rights Reserved. May not be scanned, copied or duplicated, or posted to a publicly accessible website, in whole or in part.

14. A client with the diagnosis of arthritis and congestive heart failure eats very little, adheres to a strict fluid restriction, has shortness of breath with stair climbing, and has not had a bowel movement for 2 days. The client's current vital signs are BP 136/80, P 102, R 20, T 99.2°F. The most accurate nursing diagnosis for this client would be

    a. *Deficient fluid volume* R/T fluid restriction.

    b. *Constipation* R/T poor nutritional status.

    c. *Ineffective breathing pattern* R/T congestive heart failure.

    d. none of the above.

15. Which statement is a reason why nursing informatics is improving the safety of client care?

    a. More legible medical orders

    b. Point-of-care computing

    c. Increased collaboration between health care professionals

    d. Documentation of nursing diagnoses

16. Many hospitals use interdisciplinary care plans to monitor client outcomes. Which statement best explains why novice nurses need to know nursing diagnosis and nursing process?

    a. Nursing care plans assist beginning nurses to determine the best possible nursing actions and desired client outcomes for individualized client care.

    b. Care plans assist the beginning nurse in understanding the discipline of nursing and how it relates to the care focus of other health care disciplines.

    c. Interdisciplinary care plans are used so as not to confuse nursing documentation with medical staff documentation.

    d. These plans avoid duplication of care.

17. A nursing diagnosis that identifies behaviors indicating a desire to increase well-being would be considered a(n) _____ diagnosis.

    a. actual

    b. risk

    c. health promotion

    d. wellness

© 2011 Cengage Learning. All Rights Reserved. May not be scanned, copied or duplicated, or posted to a publicly accessible website, in whole or in part.

18. The difference between a two-part nursing diagnosis statement and a three-part nursing diagnosis statement is that the three-part statement includes which additional component?

    a. Definition of the health problem

    b. Summary of medications

    c. Medical diagnosis related to the nursing problem

    d. Defining characteristics

19. The NANDA II Taxonomy organizes the NANDA-approved nursing diagnoses according to three levels, which are _____, _____, and _____.

20. The nurse is working with information cues to create appropriate nursing diagnoses for a client. Which step of the process is analogous to assembling a jigsaw puzzle?

    a. Clustering cues

    b. Interpreting cues

    c. Synthesizing cues

    d. Validating cues

Critical Thinking

21. Explain why some nurses may not like to use nursing diagnoses when planning client care.

22. Discuss why the NANDA-approved list of nursing diagnoses will never be "complete."

Activities

23. Create nursing diagnoses that could be appropriate for the following medical diagnoses:

    a. Diabetes mellitus

    b. Rape

    c. Stroke

    d. Throat cancer

    e. Appendectomy

© 2011 Cengage Learning. All Rights Reserved. May not be scanned, copied or duplicated, or posted to a publicly accessible website, in whole or in part.

24. In the clinical area, conduct an assessment on a client and determine nursing diagnoses that would be appropriate to address the client's problems. Write the diagnoses as both two-part and three-part statements. When determining a diagnosis, justify the selection by explaining what data cues and clusters were used.

25. Discuss the use of nursing diagnoses with practicing nurses. Do the nurses use nursing diagnoses? Ask why a nurse might not use nursing diagnoses.

© 2011 Cengage Learning. All Rights Reserved. May not be scanned, copied or duplicated, or posted to a publicly accessible website, in whole or in part.

Chapter 8 — Planning and Outcome Identification

1. List three elements of the planning process.

   a. _____

   b. _____

   c. _____

2. According to the ANA Standards, which is a criterion for the development of client expected outcomes?

   a. The outcome must include a time frame.

   b. The outcome must be comprehensive.

   c. The outcome must be setting specific.

   d. The outcome must be approved by an outside reviewer.

3. Match the term in the left column with its definition from the right column.

   _____ initial planning   a. An expectation to be achieved in a few days or hours

   _____ ongoing planning   b. The plan developed for the client's care on leaving the facility

   _____ discharge planning   c. The continuous updating of the client's plan of care

   _____ short-term goal   d. The plan developed as a result of the admission assessment

   _____ long-term goal   e. An expectation to be achieved in weeks or months

4. Prioritize the following nursing diagnoses from high to low priority.

   _____ *Hyperthermia*

   _____ *Risk for impaired skin integrity*

   _____ *Spiritual distress*

   _____ *Potential for fluid volume deficit*

© 2011 Cengage Learning. All Rights Reserved. May not be scanned, copied or duplicated, or posted to a publicly accessible website, in whole or in part.

5. A client tells the nurse that he would like to be shaved since he has not been so since admitted to the hospital. How should the nurse respond to this client?

    a. "I have no time to shave you today."

    b. "I will see if this can be fit into your plan of care and will let you know."

    c. "I understand your need to be shaved and will see to it that it occurs today."

    d. "Is your wife coming in today? Maybe she can shave you."

6. When determining goals, what should a short-term goal focus on?

    a. The problem

    b. The outcome

    c. The etiology

    d. The task

7. Which component is part of the task statement when writing a goal?

    a. Time limit

    b. Amount of activity

    c. Description of the performance to be followed

    d. Action verb

8. Which of the following does *not* describe a goal statement?

    a. It is measurable.

    b. It is written in current or past tense.

    c. It specifies a time frame for the task accomplishment.

    d. It is realistic for the client.

9. Which type of nursing order is "Teach the client the importance of adherence to a low-fat diet"?

    a. Health promotion

    b. Prevention

    c. Observation

    d. Treatment

© 2011 Cengage Learning. All Rights Reserved. May not be scanned, copied or duplicated, or posted to a publicly accessible website, in whole or in part.

10. Which would be an example of a client need where the nurse would call a consultation?

   a. The client is immobile and at risk for a break in skin integrity.

   b. The client has a knowledge deficit regarding ambulation with crutches on a flat surface as well as climbing stairs.

   c. The client has a Foley catheter and a primary IV infusing and is at risk for infection.

   d. The client is confused and frail with a history of falls and is at risk for injury.

11. Which portion of this goal statement is the *task statement?* "The client will ambulate the entire length of the hallway three times by Friday."

   a. The client

   b. Will ambulate

   c. The entire length of the hallway

   d. By Friday

12. A goal identified for a client is as follows: "The client will mix the two types of prescribed insulin in one syringe in preparation for injection by Tuesday." Which part of this goal states the conditions?

   a. Will mix

   b. Two types of prescribed insulin

   c. In preparation for injection

   d. By Tuesday

13. A client has the following goal: "The client will state three reasons for retaining fluid by Friday." This goal would be considered as one appropriate for a

   a. knowledge deficit.

   b. actual problem.

   c. potential problem.

   d. risk problem.

14. The nurse is selecting nursing interventions for a client's plan of care. The resources the nurse can use to assist in this process might include

   a. standardized care plans.

   b. the Internet.

   c. the nurse practice act, state board of nursing regulations, and professional standards for nursing care.

   d. interventions used for other clients.

© 2011 Cengage Learning. All Rights Reserved. May not be scanned, copied or duplicated, or posted to a publicly accessible website, in whole or in part.

15. The nurse is writing nursing orders that include the date, action verb, time frame, and signature. List what is missing from the nursing orders.

_____

16. A client is admitted with unstable BUN, creatinine, and glucose levels. The client has a history of diabetes, end-stage renal disease, and peripheral vascular disease. Which goal would be appropriate for this client?

    a. The client will plan a low-protein, 1800-calorie diabetic diet for 48 hours by Friday.

    b. The client will demonstrate effective coping by discharge.

    c. The client will be able to plan for an appropriate diet by Thursday.

    d. The client will know why it is important to follow a diet by discharge.

17. A health care organization uses standardized care plans. How should these care plans be used to meet client needs?

    a. Select the plan that most closely fits the client's needs.

    b. Edit the plan to individualize it to meet the client's needs.

    c. Include assessment in the care plan.

    d. Include the rationale for interventions in the care plan.

18. Consider the nursing diagnosis for a 1-day postop client: *Risk for infection* R/T surgical incision. Which intervention would be appropriate for this nursing diagnosis?

    a. Assess wound for signs of redness or drainage q shift.

    b. Assess IV site for inflammation or infiltration.

    c. Change Steri-Strips q shift, and assess wound.

    d. Monitor pulse rate q 4h.

19. Consider the nursing diagnosis for a client who is on bedrest: *Risk for ineffective breathing pattern* R/T stasis of secretions secondary to immobility. Which nursing intervention on the care plan was derived from the etiological portion of the nursing diagnostic statement?

    a. Offer the client a back rub q shift.

    b. Encourage client to do leg exercises q 2h.

    c. Assist client to turn, deep breathe, and cough q 2h.

    d. Suction oral secretions PRN.

© 2011 Cengage Learning. All Rights Reserved. May not be scanned, copied or duplicated, or posted to a publicly accessible website, in whole or in part.

20. Which system of standardized nursing language provides a basis to measure the effects of nursing practice on client outcomes?

    a. NIC

    b. NOC

    c. NANDA

    d. ICD-9

Critical Thinking

21. Discuss what should be done if a client has a higher priority for a nursing diagnosis than the nurse does.

22. Explain the difference between an observation nursing order and a treatment nursing order.

Activities

23. Complete the assessment of a client. Once completed, identify nursing diagnoses and then

    a. set goals.

    b. establish expected outcomes.

    c. plan interventions.

    d. write nursing orders for each intervention.

24. For the plan of care started in Question 23, access the Web link http://www.nursing.uiowa.edu/excellence/nursing_knowledge/clinical_effectiveness/documents/Label%20Definitions%20NOC%204th.pdf and choose the appropriate Nursing Outcomes Classification label for each expected outcome identified for the client.

25. For the plan of care begun in Question 23, identify rationales for each nursing intervention/order. Document the scientific source for the rationale.

© 2011 Cengage Learning. All Rights Reserved. May not be scanned, copied or duplicated, or posted to a publicly accessible website, in whole or in part.

Chapter 9   Implementation

1. At the beginning of a work shift, a nurse establishes a shift worksheet considering client care priorities. Which would be placed on the shift worksheet first?

   a. Medication administration

   b. Client assessments

   c. Care plan reviews

   d. Vital sign measurements

2. The transfer of tasks to an individual who is competent in performing these tasks is called

   a. delegation.

   b. management.

   c. validation.

   d. task segmentation.

3. Match the type of nursing management system in the left column with its definition in the right column.

   _____ functional nursing   a. The RN is the leader, LPNs care for acutely ill clients, and nursing assistants serve trays and assist with ADLs.

   _____ team nursing   b. The RN assumes responsibility for client care and coordination of care regardless of the location of the client.

   _____ primary nursing   c. Caregivers are assigned to a segment of the client care unit.

   _____ modular nursing   d. Care is divided into tasks, and each person assumes a task.

   _____ case management   e. The RN assumes responsibility for total client care.

4. Which care management system is the most costly to maintain?

   a. Team nursing

   b. Modular care

   c. Case management

   d. Primary nursing

© 2011 Cengage Learning. All Rights Reserved. May not be scanned, copied or duplicated, or posted to a publicly accessible website, in whole or in part.

5. Nursing interventions are

    a. actions that help clients achieve goals.

    b. written broadly, not specifically.

    c. exclusively independent of prescribing practitioners' orders.

    d. written as goal statements.

6. Which would *not* be a nursing intervention?

    a. Performing a thoracentesis

    b. Assisting with ADLs

    c. Discharge planning

    d. Drawing blood from a central line catheter

7. Which is considered an example of a standing prescribing practitioner's order?

    a. A protocol for indwelling urinary catheter care

    b. Hemoglobin and hematocrit 2 days postpartum on all postpartum clients

    c. The procedure for the flush of peripherally inserted central line catheters

    d. A skin care protocol for a client who is immobile

8. The nurse is determining rationales for nursing interventions. Which term best describes a rationale?

    a. Theory

    b. Pathophysiological condition

    c. Fundamental principle

    d. Nursing measure

9. The standardized nursing language that offers the profession of nursing the potential for direct reimbursement of services is

    a. NIC.

    b. NOC.

    c. NANDA.

    d. ANA.

© 2011 Cengage Learning. All Rights Reserved. May not be scanned, copied or duplicated, or posted to a publicly accessible website, in whole or in part.

10. A client tells the nurse that he does not want to have a particular intervention done. How should the nurse respond to the client?

    a. "I will tell your prescribing practitioner."

    b. "I think you should have it done."

    c. "Maybe you are ready to go home then."

    d. "You have the right to refuse any intervention."

11. The nurse is not sure about which intravenous line to use to infuse an intravenous medication. The client has several lines infusing total parental nutrition, Intralipid, and potassium chloride. What should the nurse do to ensure the medication is administered safely?

    a. Ask the prescribing practitioner.

    b. Stop one of the infusions, and use the line temporarily for the medication.

    c. Consult a resource such as an intravenous therapy policy manual, or call the pharmacy.

    d. Use any of the lines.

12. The class of nursing interventions "Electrolyte and acid-base management" falls into which domain of the Nursing Interventions Taxonomy?

    a. Physiological: Basic

    b. Physiological: Complex

    c. Safety Care

    d. Health System Care

13. The primary focus of the case manager is

    a. achieving client satisfaction.

    b. demonstrating clinical expertise.

    c. assuring services are outcome focused.

    d. developing protocol and tools for discharge.

14. Which nursing intervention is considered a skilled therapeutic intervention?

    a. Assisting a client to ambulate with a walker

    b. Feeding a client who has difficulty swallowing

    c. Bathing a client who is confused

    d. Administering a medication to a client who is hypertensive

© 2011 Cengage Learning. All Rights Reserved. May not be scanned, copied or duplicated, or posted to a publicly accessible website, in whole or in part.

15. Two tools the nursing case manager uses to evaluate a client's progress toward recovery are

    _____ and _____.

16. The nurse has completed carrying out an intervention. What should the nurse do next?

    a. Inform the prescribing practitioner that the intervention was completed.

    b. Explain the reason for the intervention to the client.

    c. Document that the intervention was completed and the client's response.

    d. Mark that the intervention was completed on the task list.

17. Which would create an opportunity for the nurse to teach a client?

    a. Medication administration

    b. Vital sign measurement

    c. Changing a wound dressing

    d. All of the above

18. When a task is delegated, the role of the nurse is to

    a. validate the skill level of the care provider.

    b. assume the task was completed as expected.

    c. allow the care provider independence during task completion.

19. List four factors a case manager would consider when planning a client's discharge.

    a. _____

    b. _____

    c. _____

    d. _____

20. The nurse is measuring a client's intake and output. This intervention would be considered

    a. teaching.

    b. supervising.

    c. therapeutic.

    d. surveillance.

© 2011 Cengage Learning. All Rights Reserved. May not be scanned, copied or duplicated, or posted to a publicly accessible website, in whole or in part.

Critical Thinking

21. Discuss the skills the nurse needs to possess to successfully implement nursing interventions.

22. Discuss the most cost-effective nursing management system that would best support an acute client care unit with 42 beds that spans two long hallways with the nurses' station located at the intersection of the two hallways. The utility rooms for supplies, medications, and wastes are also located in the center of the unit.

Activities

23. In the clinical area, determine the nursing management system used. Depending on the system, determine the following:

  a. What is the role of the registered nurse?

  b. Are licensed nurses utilized in the care area? What is their role?

  c. Are unlicensed assistive personnel used in the care area? What is their role? What tasks are they assigned?

  d. If team nursing is utilized, who provides the change-of-shift report?

24. Obtain a variety of standing orders and protocols from the clinical areas. Determine the differences between the standing orders and the protocols. Brainstorm additional sets of standing orders and/or protocols that would expedite client care.

25. A client is prescribed a new blood pressure medication. Design a teaching plan to instruct the client on how to take this medication.

26. Invite case managers and discharge planners to the classroom to discuss the role they play in client care. What challenges do they face when attempting to facilitate client discharges in a timely manner?

© 2011 Cengage Learning. All Rights Reserved. May not be scanned, copied or duplicated, or posted to a publicly accessible website, in whole or in part.

Chapter 10 Evaluation

1. Check all of the behaviors that apply to the evaluation of nursing care.

    _____ a. Establishing the initial database for a client as a result of the admission assessment

    _____ b. Juxtaposing the client's response against an expected outcome

    _____ c. Inviting the parents of a pediatric client to discuss the progress of their child toward an expected outcome

    _____ d. Interpreting a cardiac rhythm strip

    _____ e. Determining whether an objective on the care plan was achieved by the client

    _____ f. Asking the client what he or she would like to achieve as an outcome of treatment

2. Which outcome would you expect as a result of a nursing audit?

    a. Revision of the facility mission and philosophy statement

    b. Revision to the standards of care related to the prevention of falls

    c. Revision to the care plan of an individual client

    d. Revision of the job description of the unlicensed assistive personnel (UAP)

3. In which phase of the nursing process is the evaluation process reflected?

    a. Assessment and implementation

    b. Assessment and diagnosis

    c. Outcome identification and implementation

    d. Assessment, diagnosis, planning, and implementation

4. The nurse is reviewing a registered nurse job description for accuracy. The type of evaluation the nurse is conducting is a(n) _____ evaluation.

    a. structural

    b. process

    c. outcome

    d. behavioral

© 2011 Cengage Learning. All Rights Reserved. May not be scanned, copied or duplicated, or posted to a publicly accessible website, in whole or in part.

5. Which evaluation method reflects a process evaluation?

    a. The assistant manager reviews the medical records of 10 discharged clients for documentation of client response to analgesics.

    b. The division director makes rounds on all client care areas to see if nursing policies are accessible.

    c. The evening supervisor analyzes evening shift staffing patterns to ensure adequate staffing levels to meet client needs.

    d. The case manager determines whether a client's discharge goal related to knowledge deficiency has been met.

6. A client's achievement of outcomes may be evaluated by using (Select all that apply.)

    a. NIC Taxonomy.

    b. NOC Taxonomy.

    c. NANDA diagnoses.

    d. policies.

    e. Joint Commission standards.

7. Which element is an indicator of quality care?

    a. Level of client's functionality at time of discharge

    b. Prescribing practitioner satisfaction with nursing care

    c. Results of the client satisfaction survey

    d. Level of client comorbidity at time of admission

8. A prescribing practitioner asks if a client has met the expected outcome of ambulating around the unit four times each day with minimal assistance. Which primary data source should be consulted to respond to the prescribing practitioner?

    a. Client record

    b. Family

    c. Unlicensed assistive personnel

    d. Client

9. A client has not met an expected outcome. What should be done?

    a. Hold an interdisciplinary meeting.

    b. Ask the client why the goal was not met.

    c. Call a nursing consultation.

    d. Review and revise the care plan.

© 2011 Cengage Learning. All Rights Reserved. May not be scanned, copied or duplicated, or posted to a publicly accessible website, in whole or in part.

10. Registered nurses demonstrate professional accountability by

   a. obtaining advanced degrees.

   b. seeking certifications.

   c. maintaining expertise in skills.

   d. working overtime routinely.

11. Evaluation is based primarily on

   a. information retrieval and documentation.

   b. observation and communication.

   c. effective use of the nursing process.

   d. delivery of nursing care and analysis of client goals.

12. After evaluating the outcome of care, it has been determined that a goal was not met. What should occur first?

   a. Reassess the client.

   b. Formulate new nursing diagnoses.

   c. Develop new goals.

   d. Implement different nursing actions.

13. An aspect of evaluation that provides a basis for autonomy and self-governance for nursing practice is

   a. the application of agency standards.

   b. the peer evaluation process.

   c. multidisciplinary collaboration.

   d. the application of union rules to nursing practice.

14. Which statement describes evaluation?

   a. It answers questions.

   b. It is an easy process conducted by observation.

   c. It is a critical thinking activity.

   d. It is done the day of discharge.

© 2011 Cengage Learning. All Rights Reserved. May not be scanned, copied or duplicated, or posted to a publicly accessible website, in whole or in part.

15. What will be evaluated during a structure evaluation?

    a. Standards of care

    b. Policies and procedures

    c. Client's self-care abilities

    d. Client's level of wellness

16. Peer evaluation promotes professionalism and can result in two outcomes, which are either _____ and improve the quality of care or _____ and undermine morale and cohesiveness.

17. Multidisciplinary evaluations help to promote

    a. accountability.

    b. leadership.

    c. dependence.

    d. a continuum of client care.

Critical Thinking

18. Explain how the nurse's behavior can positively or negatively impact the evaluation of a client's outcomes of care.

19. Discuss the seven steps involved in the evaluation process.

Activities

20. Attend a quality improvement committee meeting or invite members of a quality improvement committee to the class. Interview the members regarding their roles in structure, process, and outcome evaluations.

21. Access the Web site http://jointcommission.org and research the most recent version of the National Patient Safety Goals. Create a nursing audit tool that can be used to evaluate whether the National Patient Safety Goal standards expected by the Joint Commission are being achieved.

© 2011 Cengage Learning. All Rights Reserved. May not be scanned, copied or duplicated, or posted to a publicly accessible website, in whole or in part.

Chapter 11 Leadership, Delegation, and Power

1. Which statement best describes the current status of nursing as a profession?

    a. Nursing is a true profession because of the existence of the American Nurses Association and the licensure needed in order to practice.

    b. Nursing has been attempting to meet the criteria of a profession since the beginning of the twentieth century.

    c. Nursing is an occupation; therefore, it is a profession.

    d. Nursing is a profession because it has a voice in legislative activity.

2. Describe two methods a registered nurse may use to maintain and communicate clinical competency.

    a. _____

    b. _____

3. To which group is a nurse accountable?

    a. The client and the client's family

    b. The nursing profession

    c. The employer

    d. All of the above

4. Match the term in the left column with its definition from the right column.

    _____ professional regulation   a. The law governing nursing practice within a state

    _____ professional standards   b. Process by which a nongovernmental agency states that an individual licensed to practice a profession has met predetermined standards set for practice

    _____ accreditation   c. The method by which states hold the individual nurse accountable for safe practice to citizens of that state

    _____ certification   d. Process by which nursing ensures that its members act in the public interest

    _____ scope of practice   e. Statements by which quality of service, practice, and education can be judged

    _____ nurse practice act   f. Legal boundaries of practice set by state statutes

    _____ licensure   g. An agency granting status to an institution that has met predetermined criteria

© 2011 Cengage Learning. All Rights Reserved. May not be scanned, copied or duplicated, or posted to a publicly accessible website, in whole or in part.

5. A nurse has minimal expertise with clients diagnosed with multiple sclerosis. What should the nurse do to maintain professional accountability when working with clients with multiple sclerosis?

    a. Refuse to provide care to clients with this diagnosis.

    b. Provide only basic care to these clients.

    c. Delegate the care of these clients to other nurses with more expertise.

    d. Attend a continuing education program to learn more about the care of clients with this diagnosis.

6. A nurse says that certification is just another way for organizations to impose limits on the practice of nursing. What is the correct response to this statement?

    a. This is true, and certification should not be supported by anyone in nursing.

    b. This is true, but some nurses like to have this credential for employment purposes.

    c. This is not true, and certification signifies a higher level of competence than is expected at the time of initial licensure.

    d. This is not true, and certification is a better credential to earn instead of having to sit for the NCLEX examination again.

7. Which statement best explains the reason for establishing the mutual recognition model for nursing licensure?

    a. The increase in the number of nurses who hold licensure in more than one state

    b. The increase in practice occurring across state lines

    c. The need to increase competency by expecting nurses to attend more continuing education programs to maintain multistate licensure

    d. The need to eliminate individual state boards of nursing and shift nursing licensure to the federal level

8. Which organization prepares students to become contributing members of the nursing profession?

    a. NSNA (National Student Nurses Association)

    b. ANA (American Nurses Association)

    c. NLN (National League for Nursing)

    d. ICN (International Council of Nurses)

9. Which organization promotes nursing accountability by establishing educational standards and surveying schools of nursing?

    a. ANA

    b. ICN

    c. Joint Commission

    d. NLN

© 2011 Cengage Learning. All Rights Reserved. May not be scanned, copied or duplicated, or posted to a publicly accessible website, in whole or in part.

10. Which of the following Standards of Professional Performance is defined as "working with others to provide client care?"

    a. Collaboration

    b. Education

    c. Research

    d. Performance Appraisal

11. List three methods the nursing profession uses to ensure accountability to the public.

    a. _____

    b. _____

    c. _____

12. By which method does a state board of nursing hold an individual accountable for safe practice?

    a. Ensuring that individuals adhere to the nursing code of ethics

    b. Developing national standards of nursing practice

    c. Requiring individuals to pass an examination that determines the minimum level of practice competency

    d. Working with the Joint Commission to establish standards for safe practice and monitoring for any breach of safe practice

13. Match the type of leadership style in the left column with an example of it from the right column.

    _____ autocratic   a. The unit manager allows an aggressive staff member to consistently dominate the staff meetings.

    _____ democratic   b. The leader of the risk management committee is directive at times while at other times lets the group problem solve.

    _____ laissez-faire   c. The case manager gives background information about the client's case to the multidisciplinary team and then invites discussion about the client's plan of care.

    _____ situational   d. The unit manager tells the staff what will be done to solve the unit's staffing problem.

14. In which style of leadership would the expected outcome be the empowerment of group members?

    a. Autocratic

    b. Democratic

    c. Laissez-faire

    d. Situational

© 2011 Cengage Learning. All Rights Reserved. May not be scanned, copied or duplicated, or posted to a publicly accessible website, in whole or in part.

15. A UAP asks the nurse if she could change a client's abdominal dressing. What should the nurse determine first before deciding to delegate this task to the UAP?

    a. Is the person competent to do the task?

    b. Can this task be delegated?

    c. Will the delegation of the task put the client at risk?

    d. What are the prescribing practitioner's orders about the abdominal dressing?

16. A graduate nurse, just completing her first 2 months of orientation, has been assigned to do charge in the night shift. Which of the "four rights of delegation" does this situation involve?

    a. Right task

    b. Right person

    c. Right communication

    d. Right feedback

17. The nurse manager is reviewing performance standards in order to complete a nurse's annual performance review. Which management function is the nurse manager utilizing?

    a. Decision making

    b. Controlling

    c. Planning

    d. Organizing

18. Which reflects positive mentor behavior?

    a. An experienced staff nurse readily offers the answer to any question.

    b. A unit manager allows a novice nurse to find a solution to a clinical problem.

    c. The chairperson of a newly formed committee allows the committee members to find their own direction.

    d. A nursing instructor offers to coach a nursing student in exchange for babysitting services.

19. There is one nurse who knows how to use a device that places pressure on a blood vessel after a cardiac catheterization. What type of power does this nurse have?

    a. Legitimate

    b. Referent

    c. Expert

    d. Reward

© 2011 Cengage Learning. All Rights Reserved. May not be scanned, copied or duplicated, or posted to a publicly accessible website, in whole or in part.

20. Of the following client activities, select those that can be performed by a UAP.

  _____   a. Maintaining an intravenous line

  _____   b. Ambulating a client

  _____   c. Making a bed

  _____   d. Removing sutures

  _____   e. Measuring intake and output

  _____   f. Passing medications

Critical Thinking

21. Explain the purpose of the American Nurses Association, including why a nurse would want to become a member of this organization.

22. Discuss the "politics" of nursing.

Activities

23. Access the American Nurses Association Web site at http://nursingworld.org. Under the "Especially for You" area (on the left), click on the Student Nurses link. Consider the advantages of becoming a student member of the ANA. List the benefits associated with becoming a student member.

24. Attend a committee meeting at school or for a community organization. Study the behavior of the committee chairperson. What type of leadership style is the committee chairperson demonstrating? List examples of the leadership style. Discuss the committee meeting and chairperson's behavior in small groups.

25. Access the American Nurses Credentialing Center at http://www.nursecredentialing.org. Research the different types of certification programs available to nurses. Identify one certification of interest to you, and list the reasons why it would be beneficial to earn this credential.

© 2011 Cengage Learning. All Rights Reserved. May not be scanned, copied or duplicated, or posted to a publicly accessible website, in whole or in part.

Chapter 12 Legal and Ethical Responsibilities

1. Which mandate is the result of state administrative law action?

   a. Controlled Substances Act

   b. Nurse Practice Act

   c. Social Security Act

   d. National Labor Relations Act

2. Match the term in the left column with its definition in the right column.

   _____ malpractice   a. Person being sued

   _____ negligence   b. Breach of duty

   _____ plaintiff   c. Wrongful conduct by a professional

   _____ defendant   d. Party seeking damages

   _____ testimony   e. Written or verbal evidence given by an expert in an area

3. Place the following elements for the proof of liability in the proper sequence.

   _____ Injury is established.

   _____ There was an obligation created by law, contract, or any voluntary action.

   _____ A cause and effect is established linking the breach of duty to the injury.

   _____ An act of omission or commission caused a breach of duty.

4. Under which condition is it legal to apply restraints?

   a. When a client is confused

   b. When a client is in danger of harming himself or harming others

   c. When a client is agitated

   d. When a client is threatening to leave the hospital against medical advice (AMA)

© 2011 Cengage Learning. All Rights Reserved. May not be scanned, copied or duplicated, or posted to a publicly accessible website, in whole or in part.

5. Which action by a nurse demonstrates an understanding of a client's right to privacy? The nurse

   a. checks on the client using the intercom.

   b. ensures the noise level in a client's room is kept to a minimum.

   c. knocks before entering a room.

   d. limits the visitors of a seriously ill client.

6. A nurse is overheard in the elevator discussing a neighbor, saying he was recently diagnosed with AIDS. This nurse can be held liable for

   a. slander.

   b. libel.

   c. fraud.

   d. negligence.

7. Which type of health concern is covered by the Americans with Disabilities Act (ADA)?

   a. Psychiatric disorders

   b. Smoking

   c. Skin disorders

   d. Seasonal allergies

8. To what standard would a nurse be held when responding to an emergency in the community?

   a. By how a reasonable and prudent caregiver would have acted in the same situation.

   b. The nurse has full immunity from litigation.

   c. By the standards set forth in the local community hospital for emergency care.

   d. The nurse has full immunity as long as no money is accepted for the care rendered during the emergency.

9. A client refuses an injection; however, the nurse administers it against the client's will. Of which charge can the nurse can be found guilty?

   a. Assault and battery

   b. False imprisonment

   c. Libel

   d. Slander

© 2011 Cengage Learning. All Rights Reserved. May not be scanned, copied or duplicated, or posted to a publicly accessible website, in whole or in part.

10. A client who has received three doses of a narcotic analgesic continues to complain of pain. A similar incident occurred a few days ago. The nurse suspects that the narcotics are being signed out but not administered. What should the nurse do?

   a.   Do nothing.

   b.   Monitor the situation.

   c.   Report the nurse who is signing out the narcotics to the nursing supervisor.

   d.   Report the nurse who is signing out the narcotics to the state board of nursing.

11. What should a nurse do regarding liability insurance?

   a.   Do nothing since the employer has this insurance.

   b.   Do nothing, but keep an attorney on retainer in the event of a lawsuit.

   c.   Buy the same insurance as the employer.

   d.   Purchase individual insurance after validating the company's reputation.

12. List four areas in nursing practice where nurses are at legal risk.

   a.   _____

   b.   _____

   c.   _____

   d.   _____

13. A safety issue in health care is the prevention of medication errors. The most common type of medication errors are all of the following *except*

   a.   administering to the incorrect client.

   b.   giving the incorrect dosage.

   c.   giving the incorrect drug.

   d.   not administering the medication.

14. What should the nurse do to reduce the risk of liability when a client falls?

   a.   Document the incident carefully on an incident report form.

   b.   Chart the facts about the fall, the client's condition, and follow-up care.

   c.   Do not document anything about the fall.

   d.   Change assignments after the fall.

© 2011 Cengage Learning. All Rights Reserved. May not be scanned, copied or duplicated, or posted to a publicly accessible website, in whole or in part.

15. The nurse is not sure about an order written for a medication for a client. What should the nurse do?

    a. Administer the medication.

    b. Ask another nurse about the order.

    c. Contact the prescribing practitioner for clarification.

    d. Ignore the order and leave it for the next nurse to administer.

16. The nurse watches a client sign a consent form for surgery. Which of the following is the nurse witnessing?

    a. The client understands the procedure.

    b. The client signed the form.

    c. The client realizes the risks of the procedure.

    d. The client agrees to receive blood during the procedure.

17. Informed consent indicates the client

    a. is mentally competent.

    b. understands all the implications surrounding a proposed intervention.

    c. is providing voluntary agreement.

    d. signed a witness consent form.

18. In which document would a nurse seek to learn the name of the responsible person appointed by the client to make health care decisions for that client when the client is unable to make his or her own health care decisions?

    a. Durable power of attorney

    b. Living will

    c. Advance care medical directive

    d. General consent form

19. Risk management programs are aimed at decreasing the risk of financial loss to the

    a. prescribing practitioner.

    b. agency.

    c. prescribing practitioner and nurse.

    d. agency, prescribing practitioner, and nurse.

© 2011 Cengage Learning. All Rights Reserved. May not be scanned, copied or duplicated, or posted to a publicly accessible website, in whole or in part.

20. Which is the purpose of DNR prescribing practitioner's orders?

    a. To document the terminal nature of the client's condition

    b. To allow an alternative to the universal standing order to provide cardiopulmonary resuscitation to all clients

    c. To provide an opportunity for the client, family, and caregivers to discuss the nature of the client's condition and the best possible course of action if the client has a cardiac arrest

    d. To provide legal protection for nurses who believe a client should not be resuscitated

21. Match the term in the left column with its definition from the right column.

    _____ ethics   a. The personal beliefs held by an individual that reflect religion or tradition

    _____ morals   b. What a person considers of worth, indirectly impacting behavior

    _____ values   c. The application of ethical principles to health care

    _____ ethical principles d. Codes that direct or govern our actions

    _____ bioethics   e. The branch of philosophy that concerns the distinction of right and wrong on the basis of a body of knowledge

22. Conducting oneself ethically as a nurse embodies respect for human rights, the right to dignity, and the right to be treated with respect. These values are included in

    a. values and teaching.

    b. International Council of Nurses *Code for Nurses*.

    c. American Nurses Association *Code for Nurses*.

    d. Canadian Nurses Association *Code of Ethics*.

23. The Nightingale Pledge states that while clients are under the care of a nurse, the nurse is to do no harm to the client. Which of the following ethical principles does this represent?

    a. Justice

    b. Nonmaleficence

    c. Fidelity

    d. Beneficence

© 2011 Cengage Learning. All Rights Reserved. May not be scanned, copied or duplicated, or posted to a publicly accessible website, in whole or in part.

24. Match the ethical principle in the left column with an appropriate example from the right column.

    _____ autonomy

    _____ nonmaleficence

    _____ beneficence

    _____ justice

    _____ veracity

    _____ fidelity

    a. The nurse represents the client's viewpoint accurately during the interdisciplinary conference.

    b. A client is asked to sign an informed consent form by a prescribing practitioner.

    c. The nurse signs for a wasted narcotic only after she sees it being discarded.

    d. The nurse triple checks the medication for right medication and right dose.

    e. The nurse considers whether a client should be physically restrained.

    f. The client assignments on the unit are equally divided among the nurses.

25. A client does not want to have a medication because it is not supported by the client's religious beliefs. What should the nurse do?

    a. Persuade the client to take the medication.

    b. Refuse to be the nurse for the client.

    c. Suggest the client sign out of the hospital.

    d. Support the client.

26. List three frequently occurring ethical dilemmas in health care.

    a. _____

    b. _____

    c. _____

27. Which is *not* included in the American Hospital Association (1972) "Patient's Bill of Rights"?

    a. The client has the right to considerate and respectful care.

    b. The client has the right to make decisions about the plan of care.

    c. The client has the right to have an advance directive concerning treatment.

    d. The client has the right to sign a release of responsibility and leave the hospital at any time.

© 2011 Cengage Learning. All Rights Reserved. May not be scanned, copied or duplicated, or posted to a publicly accessible website, in whole or in part.

28. The home care nurse sits with a client to develop a plan of care for medications and activities of daily living. Which client right is the nurse preserving?

   a. The right to make decisions regarding her care

   b. Her right to be involved in the treatment process

   c. The right to be treated with dignity and respect

   d. All of the above

29. In which step in the ethical decision-making process would the ethical dilemma be stated?

   a. Determination of claims and identification of parties

   b. Problem identification

   c. Generation of alternatives

   d. Assessing the outcome of moral actions

30. Which best defines an ethical dilemma?

   a. A conflict between two or more ethical principles

   b. A conflict between the interests of two or more parties in the care of an individual

   c. A choice between two equally satisfactory alternatives

   d. A choice between the desired action of the nurse and the client

31. An ethical dilemma is being studied. At the conclusion of this study, what is the expected outcome?

   a. A clear right decision

   b. A clear wrong decision

   c. A decision that is the most beneficial according to the circumstances

   d. A decision that uses the least amount of resources

32. Match the term in the left column with its definition from the right column.

   _____ euthanasia   a. Taking deliberate action that hastens a client's death

   _____ active euthanasia   b. The omission of an action that would prolong a client's life

   _____ passive euthanasia   c. A health care professional providing the client with the means to end his or her own life

   _____ assisted suicide   d. The deliberate ending of a life as a human action

© 2011 Cengage Learning. All Rights Reserved. May not be scanned, copied or duplicated, or posted to a publicly accessible website, in whole or in part.

33. What is the ANA position on the participation of nurses in active euthanasia?

    a. Participation is in violation of nursing's ethical code.

    b. Participation is sanctioned only when the circumstances clearly warrant such action.

    c. Nursing's ethical code stands in support of active euthanasia.

    d. Participation is according to each individual nurse's decision.

34. Which government level provides protection for whistle-blowers? (Select all that apply.)

    a. Federal

    b. State

    c. County

    d. City

35. Which behavior is unethical and illegal?

    a. Taking narcotics from the narcotic cabinet for your own use

    b. Assisting a prescribing practitioner in an abortion clinic to perform an abortion

    c. Allowing a gay (homosexual) AIDS client to sleep with his partner in the hospital

    d. Giving out client information over the telephone to a spouse

36. The husband of a client recovering from bowel surgery for cancer asks that the diagnosis of cancer be withheld from the client. Which ethical principles are in conflict with the husband's request?

    a. Veracity and beneficence

    b. Veracity and nonmaleficence

    c. Justice and beneficence

    d. Fidelity and justice

Critical Thinking

37. A nurse is sued for malpractice after making an error. The nurse's friend is considered an expert witness for the case. Should the nurse's friend accept the expert witness role or decline?

38. There are sufficient staff nurses available to cover the care needs for a client area. One nurse, however, must accompany a client off of the unit, which will leave the unit understaffed for 4 hours of the shift. What should be done?

© 2011 Cengage Learning. All Rights Reserved. May not be scanned, copied or duplicated, or posted to a publicly accessible website, in whole or in part.

Activities

39.   Research recent cases of malpractice. Study the case to determine the duty, breach of duty, injury, and causation. Discuss the case in small groups.

40.   Invite an attorney who specializes in malpractice cases to come to the class to discuss the different types of cases that he or she represents. Ask the attorney (in advance) to discuss the role of the nurse as an expert witness.

41.   Research the nursing role of legal nurse consultant. What is the function of this role? What education is needed? Are there any regulations or certifications required for this role?

© 2011 Cengage Learning. All Rights Reserved. May not be scanned, copied or duplicated, or posted to a publicly accessible website, in whole or in part.

Chapter 13 Documentation and Informatics

1. It is acceptable to use abbreviations in the medical record if the abbreviation is

   a. a standard prescribing practitioner communication.

   b. American Medical Association approved.

   c. recognized by the Joint Commission.

   d. approved by the faculty's written policies.

2. Which of the following best describes nursing informatics?

   a. Familiarity with the use of personal computers

   b. Ability to recognize when information is needed

   c. Use of information and computer technology to support nursing practice

   d. Management and processing of information with the assistance of computers

3. Which is the best defense of a nurse during a malpractice lawsuit?

   a. Depositions by fellow nurses

   b. The client record

   c. Character witnesses

   d. Personal anecdotal notes

4. Which statement best describes the information contained in the consultation sheet found in the medical record?

   a. It contains medical orders and the treatment plan.

   b. It contains a record of the client's vital signs.

   c. It contains a record of the history and physical examination conducted by the attending prescribing practitioner.

   d. It contains a request for the services of other practitioners.

© 2011 Cengage Learning. All Rights Reserved. May not be scanned, copied or duplicated, or posted to a publicly accessible website, in whole or in part.

5. A form in the medical record provides information about the client's wishes regarding life-sustaining procedures if the client becomes unable to make these decisions. This form is a(n)

    a. durable power of attorney for health care.

    b. advance directive.

    c. informed consent.

    d. incident form.

6. Which statement best interprets the signature of an informed consent form by a nurse as witness to the client's signature?

    a. The client understands the procedure written on the consent form.

    b. The prescribing practitioner has explained the procedure to the client.

    c. The client is, in fact, the client and is competent to make a decision.

    d. The nurse was assigned to the client at the time of obtaining the informed consent.

7. Which approach to nursing care and documentation is used in a nursing information system?

    a. Nursing process and protocols

    b. Protocols and spreadsheets

    c. Spreadsheets and flow sheets

    d. SOAP and protocols

8. Which type of data is considered personal health information?

    a. Written communication

    b. Verbal communication

    c. Electronically transmitted information

    d. All of the above

9. What should be done if an error is made while documenting on a medical record?

    a. Erase the mistake and write over it.

    b. Scratch it out so it is completely obliterated.

    c. Cross it out and go on with the recording.

    d. Draw one line through it, and sign and date the correction.

© 2011 Cengage Learning. All Rights Reserved. May not be scanned, copied or duplicated, or posted to a publicly accessible website, in whole or in part.

10.   Which organization approves abbreviations and symbols for use in a medical record?

   a.   ANA

   b.   AMA

   c.   NANDA

   d.   The health care organization

11.   A nurse is logged into the computer system for documenting client care but has been called to assist in a client room. What should the nurse do?

   a.   Do nothing.

   b.   Turn off the computer monitor.

   c.   Log off of the system.

   d.   Disconnect the keyboard.

12.   Match the method of documentation in the left column with its example or definition from the right column.

   _____   narrative charting   a.   SOAP note entries are made in the medical record.

   _____   problem-oriented   b.   Saves documentation time, increases legibility, and facilitates the statistical analysis of data

   _____   PIE charting   c.   Flow sheets are used extensively; deviations from preestablished norms are documented.

   _____   focus charting   d.   Uses a chronological, storytelling format

   _____   charting by exception   e.   Charting uses a columnar format within the progress notes to distinguish it from other recordings in the narrative notes

   _____   computerized documentation   f.   Incorporates the ongoing plan of care into the daily charting

13.   The nurse has completed documenting care for a client and is prepared to report off to the next shift nurse. What should the nurse do if the client has any changes since the last documentation?

   a.   Add the change to the documentation.

   b.   Report the change during the change-of-shift report.

   c.   Tell the charge nurse about the change.

   d.   Ask the oncoming shift nurse to document the change.

© 2011 Cengage Learning. All Rights Reserved. May not be scanned, copied or duplicated, or posted to a publicly accessible website, in whole or in part.

14. When the nurse enters a client's room, the client states, "I am afraid of everything that is happening to me. What if someone makes a mistake?" Which statement best describes how this information should be documented?

    a. Client is highly anxious.

    b. Client thinks someone is making mistakes.

    c. Client is paranoid.

    d. Client states: "I'm afraid of everything that is happening to me. What if someone makes a mistake?"

15. Which nurse's note entry in the medical record is most accurate?

    a. Client is able to deep breathe and cough without difficulty.

    b. Client performs deep breathing and coughing exercises independently; cough is nonproductive.

    c. Client assisted with deep breathing and coughing (DB&C) exercises, expectorating small amounts of clear sputum. Lung sounds clear after DB&C activity.

    d. Client states deep breathing and coughing exercises are painful.

16. Which of the following uses telecommunication technologies and computers to exchange health care information and provide client services at another location?

    a. Internet

    b. Telehealth

    c. Telephone

    d. Personal data assistant

17. Which of the following is a necessary element in order for computerized documentation systems in health care agencies to demonstrate the quality, effectiveness, and value of nursing service?

    a. A standardized nursing language

    b. Standardized databases

    c. A final version of the nursing taxonomy

    d. Nurses who are able to improve client care delivery systems

© 2011 Cengage Learning. All Rights Reserved. May not be scanned, copied or duplicated, or posted to a publicly accessible website, in whole or in part.

18. Which is the most accurate entry on the prescribing practitioner's order sheet by a nurse after taking a telephone order from a prescribing practitioner?

    a. Give Lasix 40 mg IVP now
        T.O. Dr. Donohue/Mary Smith R.N.

    b. Verapamil 5 mg IVP stat
        Dr. Jones/Mary Smith R.N.

    c. Dulcolax tablets for constipation
        Dr. Cordovan/Mary Smith R.N.

    d. Tylenol 650 mg q 4–6h PRN for headache
        Mary Smith R.N.

19. It is recommended that nurses document a client incident of a fall carefully on the client record. Which of the following is the correct rationale for this?

    a. Falls are costly to treat.

    b. Falls are the main reason nurses are sued.

    c. The data are used by risk managers to identify factors that create risk for falls in a client population in a facility.

    d. The documentation assists the prescribing practitioner with diagnosing and treating the client's condition after the fall.

20. Which documentation system would the nurse be expected to use to document a variance from an expected outcome?

    a. Narrative charting

    b. Charting by exception

    c. Critical pathway

    d. Nursing care Kardex

Critical Thinking

21. Discuss how computers are used in nursing and what skills are needed by the nurse.

22. Explain how the use of telehealth impacts the cost of providing client care.

© 2011 Cengage Learning. All Rights Reserved. May not be scanned, copied or duplicated, or posted to a publicly accessible website, in whole or in part.

Activities

23. Using the Criteria for Evaluating Validity of Information, research Web sites on the following topics:

    a. Diabetes

    b. Heart disease

    c. Asthma

    Generate a list of Web sites that meet most or all of the criteria.

24. Invite nurses who work in the telehealth industry to the class to discuss their role as a nurse. What are the challenges? What are the opportunities? What training did they receive to transition from providing direct client care to providing care through the use of telecommunication technology?

25. Access the American Academy of Ambulatory Care Nursing Web site at http://www.aaacn.org/cgi-bin/ WebObjects/AAACNMain. Research the information provided on telehealth. Discuss why telehealth is included within the ambulatory care nursing specialty and not another specialty.

© 2011 Cengage Learning. All Rights Reserved. May not be scanned, copied or duplicated, or posted to a publicly accessible website, in whole or in part.

Chapter 14   Nursing, Healing, and Caring

1. Of the following behaviors, check which behaviors display a nurse caring for a client.

    ____ a.   Responding in a compassionate manner

    ____ b.   Anticipating a client need

    ____ c.   Responding to a client who is fearful

    ____ d.   Calling a client "hon" or "dearie"

    ____ e.   Providing preprocedural information

    ____ f.   Delaying the response to a call light

    ____ g.   Focusing attention on the treatment, not on the client

2. Care that is humanistic, emphasizing the client's individuality, counteracts which of the following processes that could occur during hospitalization?

    a. Depersonalization

    b. Oppression

    c. Empowerment

    d. Adaptation

3. Performing nursing interventions in a caring manner promotes a(n) _____ environment.

    a. empathic

    b. healing

    c. warm

    d. nonjudgmental

4. Write in the appropriate relationship type, *social* or *therapeutic*, on the lines provided.

    _____ spontaneous

    _____ communication is planned

    _____ based on mutual interests

    _____ each participant expects to be liked by the other

    _____ has clear boundaries

© 2011 Cengage Learning. All Rights Reserved. May not be scanned, copied or duplicated, or posted to a publicly accessible website, in whole or in part.

5. One trait unique to nursing involves the commitment to helping the client. This trait is considered

   a. empathy.

   b. sympathy.

   c. trust.

   d. intentionality.

6. In which phase of the nurse-client relationship would the nurse expect the client to exhibit testing behaviors?

   a. Orientation

   b. Working

   c. Termination

   d. Therapeutic

7. A nurse answers the questions of a new mother regarding newborn care at home. In which phase of the nurse-client relationship would this occur?

   a. Orientation

   b. Working

   c. Termination

   d. Therapeutic

8. Which nurse theorist believes that caring is communicated through actions?

   a. Watson

   b. Leininger

   c. Benner

   d. Maslow

9. Match the characteristic of therapeutic relationships in the left column with its definition from the right column.

   _____ catharsis   a. A connection between two people based on mutual trust

   _____ rapport   b. The process of "getting things off one's chest"

   _____ empathy   c. Acting on the behalf of the client

   _____ advocacy   d. The perception of the situation as the client perceives it

© 2011 Cengage Learning. All Rights Reserved. May not be scanned, copied or duplicated, or posted to a publicly accessible website, in whole or in part.

10. What can a nurse do to communicate a sense of caring to a client?

    a. Touch

    b. Talk

    c. Listen

    d. Ask questions

11. The therapeutic tool of the nurse where the nurse remains physically with the client is referred to as

    _____.

12. Which behavior by a nurse would foster trust?

    a. Hurriedly checking an IV site and administering the IV medication

    b. Sitting down and making frequent eye contact during a client interview

    c. Changing a client's dressing while talking to a coworker

    d. Not divulging the client's blood pressure when the client asks for this information

13. What can the nurse do to assess a client's sense of humor?

    a. Tell a joke and see if the client laughs.

    b. Do nothing since humor cannot be assessed.

    c. Observe the client to see if he or she smiles.

    d. Evaluate the client for the use of jokes or types of humor expressed by the client.

14. Match the essential behavior of trust in the left column with an example of it from the right column.

    _____ honesty   a. Providing privacy

    _____ consistency   b. Following through on a promise

    _____ respect   c. Maintaining confidentiality

15. What characteristic is being demonstrated by the nurse who is able to establish priorities to address unexpected events that require immediate action?

    a. Nonjudgmental care

    b. Flexibility

    c. Humor

    d. Risk taking

© 2011 Cengage Learning. All Rights Reserved. May not be scanned, copied or duplicated, or posted to a publicly accessible website, in whole or in part.

16. In which role is a nurse functioning when a client is helped to increase coping skills?

    a. Caregiver

    b. Teacher

    c. Resource person

    d. Counselor

17. The nurse who instructs a client about medications, diet, and exercise to manage heart disease is ultimately doing what for the client?

    a. Reducing the possibility of the onset of long-term disease

    b. Helping the client lose weight

    c. Empowering the client

    d. Encouraging the client to reduce health care costs

18. What is the goal of transcultural nursing?

    a. To provide health care within the context of the client's culture

    b. To provide expert care to clients of different cultures

    c. To recognize cultural differences

    d. To learn about the health care expectations of clients of different cultures

19. Which of the following is a nurse behavior during the orientation phase of the therapeutic relationship?

    a. Establish confidentiality parameters

    b. Support realistic problem solving

    c. Problem solve

    d. Client involvement

20. The nurse deliberately plans actions and approaches the relationship with a client with a specific goal in mind before interacting with the client. This activity is considered

    a. assessing.

    b. planning.

    c. sympathizing.

    d. therapeutic use of self.

© 2011 Cengage Learning. All Rights Reserved. May not be scanned, copied or duplicated, or posted to a publicly accessible website, in whole or in part.

Critical Thinking

21. Contrast Watson's theory of human caring with Benner's theory of novice to expert in regard to caring in nursing.

22. Discuss the characteristics of a therapeutic relationship.

23. Explain the concept of active listening.

Activities

24. Using the Internet or other resources, identify examples in the media in which humor is used in association with a health care issue. Examples can include sitcoms, movies, print, and magazine articles. Discuss the examples with others in the class.

25. Invite a panel of registered nurses to the class to discuss the roles they play when providing client care. Have questions prepared to guide the nurses into giving specific examples of the roles. Ask the nurses which roles are the most challenging and rewarding. Are any of the roles difficult to perform and why?

26. Practice empathetic responses to the following client comments:

    a. "My husband drinks and beats me at least once a month."

    b. "I have cancer and do not want any treatment whatsoever."

    c. "My mother-in-law wants to move in with my family, but she is very ill and I can't do everything that she needs done for her health."

    d. "I have so much back pain that the only thing that helps is a narcotic."

    e. "It hurts to move, so I don't move very much."

    f. "Every doctor and nurse is the same—all you do is ask the same questions over and over again. Doesn't anyone talk to each other?"

    g. "I do not want any more tests. The doctors are trying to find something wrong with me so they can bill my insurance company."

© 2011 Cengage Learning. All Rights Reserved. May not be scanned, copied or duplicated, or posted to a publicly accessible website, in whole or in part.

Chapter 15 Communication

1. The purpose of communication is to

    a. convey information to others.

    b. establish and maintain meaningful relationships.

    c. assess clients.

    d. provide feedback to the sender of a message.

2. Match the component of the communication process in the left column with the definition of the term in the right column.

    _____ sender   a. Can be verbal or nonverbal

    _____ message   b. Generates messages

    _____ channel   c. Is received as a reaction to a message

    _____ receiver   d. Intercepts messages

    _____ feedback   e. Can be auditory, visual, or kinesthetic

3. Match the type of personal space in the left column with a therapeutic example from the right column.

    _____ intimate distance   a. Teaching a diabetic education class

    _____ personal distance   b. Giving an injection

    _____ social distance   c. Client demonstration of tube feeding

4. Which of the following best explains the importance of validating communication?

    a. Many clients with whom a nurse interacts are cognitively impaired.

    b. It assists a client with clarifying thoughts.

    c. Eye contact does not send the same message from culture to culture.

    d. Perceptions influence the interpretation of a message.

© 2011 Cengage Learning. All Rights Reserved. May not be scanned, copied or duplicated, or posted to a publicly accessible website, in whole or in part.

5. A client tells the nurse that she is "confused about what is happening with me." How should the nurse respond to this client?

    a. "Why are you confused?"

    b. "Have you been given confusing information?"

    c. "Everyone has periods of confusion when in the hospital."

    d. "What are you feeling confused about?"

6. Which is a characteristic of effective feedback? It is

    a. general vs. specific.

    b. independent of time.

    c. best delivered in a small-group setting.

    d. clear and unambiguous.

7. When assessing a client's communication, the nurse assesses for congruence between the verbal and nonverbal messages the client conveys. What does congruence mean?

    a. The verbal and nonverbal messages match.

    b. The verbal and nonverbal messages do not match.

    c. The client is predominantly communicating using nonverbal cues.

    d. The client is predominantly using words to communicate.

8. All the following are barriers to effective communication *except*

    a. self-disclosure.

    b. inattentive listening.

    c. medical jargon.

    d. active listening.

9. Match the type of group in the left column with the example from the right column.

    _____ self-help group   a. Committee to study needlestick injuries

    _____ therapeutic group   b. Alcoholics Anonymous

    _____ therapy group   c. Eating disorders group

    _____ task group   d. Lifestyle change group (to reverse coronary artery disease)

© 2011 Cengage Learning. All Rights Reserved. May not be scanned, copied or duplicated, or posted to a publicly accessible website, in whole or in part.

10. A client thanks the nurse for "showing" how to fill an insulin syringe but asks if there are any printed instructions. The nurse realizes that the client's dominant communication channel most likely is

    a. visual.

    b. auditory.

    c. kinesthetic.

    d. perceptual.

11. Match the principle of therapeutic interactions in the left column with its rationale in the right column.

    _____ timeliness   a. Anxiety influences interaction

    _____ privacy   b. Allows the client to discuss problems and needs

    _____ comfort   c. Provides for confidentiality

    _____ client focus   d. Allows for discussion about troublesome events or situations

    _____ focus on client feelings   e. Ensures the client's attention during the interview

    _____ awareness of nurse's anxiety   f. Eliminates distractions

12. Which behavior of a nurse indicates to a client that the nurse is actively listening?

    a. The nurse's lips are pursed.

    b. The nurse is shifting around in the chair.

    c. The nurse makes eye contact.

    d. The nurse changes the subject frequently.

13. The nurse is caring for a client within the personal distance zone. Which action is best conducted in this zone?

    a. Administering a massage

    b. Making a bed

    c. Providing a therapeutic response to the client

    d. Hanging an intravenous solution

© 2011 Cengage Learning. All Rights Reserved. May not be scanned, copied or duplicated, or posted to a publicly accessible website, in whole or in part.

14. A nurse says, "Tell me about what concerns you most today." This request is an example of which communication technique?

    a. Broad opening statement

    b. Reflection

    c. Focusing

    d. Restating

15. The client states, "I feel so angry when my husband refuses to come to the hospital and stay with me." Which would be the best approach when the client conveys anger?

    a. Reassure the client her husband loves her.

    b. Tell her he is probably afraid of hospitals.

    c. State "My husband wouldn't come either."

    d. Explore the client's anger with her.

16. The mother of a client states that medication prescribed for a rash on her son is not working. The nurse responds, "You sound frustrated." The nurse's response is an example of which communication technique?

    a. Focusing

    b. Exploring

    c. Restating

    d. Reflection

17. A client tells the nurse that she has breathing problems after a surgical procedure and wants to know if she should worry about it. How should the nurse respond to this client?

    a. "I'm sure everything will work out. Not everyone recovers at the same rate."

    b. "No, I don't think so."

    c. "Let me look at your chart. I'll be right back. Maybe the prescribing practitioner has written something in the chart that will be of help."

    d. "Can you tell me more about your breathing problems? Describe them for me."

© 2011 Cengage Learning. All Rights Reserved. May not be scanned, copied or duplicated, or posted to a publicly accessible website, in whole or in part.

18. The nurse notes that a client is sitting on the side of the bed in a slumped posture. What does this posture convey to the nurse?

    a. Anxiety

    b. Interest

    c. Depressed

    d. Rejection

19. A client with diabetes is seen eating chocolate, appears embarrassed, and comments on the taste of the candy. How should the nurse respond to this client?

    a. "You know you shouldn't be eating those. They are not good for you."

    b. "You did the right thing by stopping. Candy is bad for you."

    c. "I noticed you seemed embarrassed when you saw me. Would you like to talk about how you are feeling?"

    d. "Would you like to review what foods are part of your diabetic diet?"

20. The nurse is sitting with a client, with a hand on the client's shoulder. Which element of therapeutic communication is the nurse demonstrating?

    a. Caring

    b. Validation

    c. Honesty

    d. Empathy

21. The nurse is communicating with a client through the use of an interpreter. What should the nurse do to facilitate caring and trust with the client?

    a. Talk to the translator.

    b. Speak directly to the client.

    c. Look at the translator.

    d. Talk with the translator outside of the client's room.

© 2011 Cengage Learning. All Rights Reserved. May not be scanned, copied or duplicated, or posted to a publicly accessible website, in whole or in part.

22. The nurse is caring for a client recovering from a stroke. The client, who cannot ambulate and has a pressure ulcer on her sacrum, says to the nurse, "I cannot walk and need help with everything. What is going to become of me?" How should the nurse respond to this client?

    a. "I'll leave a message for your prescribing practitioner, so when she comes in she can talk about your progress."

    b. "It sounds like you are depressed. We can talk about it later."

    c. "You sound afraid for the future. If you want to talk about it, I would like to hear about it."

    d. "Let me finish with this dressing and I'll get you fixed up and you will feel better."

23. A client is demonstrating difficulty naming objects and places. The nurse realizes the client is exhibiting which type of aphasia?

    a. Broca's

    b. Wernicke's

    c. Conduction

    d. Anomic

24. Which of the following skills is the foundation of therapeutic communication?

    a. Active listening

    b. Validation

    c. Interviewing

    d. Restating

25. A client is unconscious after the rupture of a cerebral aneurysm. What assumption should the nurse make when communicating with this client?

    _____

    _____

    _____

© 2011 Cengage Learning. All Rights Reserved. May not be scanned, copied or duplicated, or posted to a publicly accessible website, in whole or in part.

Critical Thinking

26.   Explain the concept of group dynamics.

27.   Discuss the situations in which a nurse should use touch with caution.

Activities

28.   Break into small groups. Provide one member of each group with ear plugs. Conduct a conversation in the group, and determine if the person with the ear plugs is able to follow the conversation. What did the person with the ear plugs hear? What was distorted?

29.   Plan for everyone to wear a specific type of artifact to the class. Each artifact should be discussed as to its significance to the person and why it was chosen to be worn.

30.   Arrange the class in small groups. Notice where each person selects to sit. Analyze if the seat chosen had any particular meaning to the person or to the group. What did the seat chosen communicate to the group?

31.   Attend a committee meeting, and analyze where everyone sits in the room. Where did the committee chairperson sit? Who sat nearest to the door? Who did the most talking during the meeting, and where did this person sit?

© 2011 Cengage Learning. All Rights Reserved. May not be scanned, copied or duplicated, or posted to a publicly accessible website, in whole or in part.

Chapter 16   Health and Wellness Promotion

1. Match the term in the left column with its definition from the right column.

   _____ health

   _____ illness

   _____ wellness

   _____ homeostasis

   _____ adaptation

   _____ high-level wellness

   a. A process through which a person seeks to maintain an equilibrium that promotes stability and comfort

   b. The process by which a person adjusts to achieve homeostasis

   c. Functioning to one's maximum health potential

   d. Optimal level of functioning

   e. Equilibrium among psychological, physiological, sociocultural, intellectual, and spiritual needs

   f. Failure of adaptive responses that results in an impairment of functional abilities

2. A client has unmet physiological needs. Which unmet need would be addressed as the highest priority?

   a. Hunger

   b. Sadness

   c. Learning deficit

   d. Sense of purpose

3. Which of the following theoretical perspectives on health would a nurse be operating through when he or she assists a person with the use of health-promoting activities?

   a. Dunn

   b. Pender

   c. Bandura

   d. Rosenstock

© 2011 Cengage Learning. All Rights Reserved. May not be scanned, copied or duplicated, or posted to a publicly accessible website, in whole or in part.

4. List three nursing actions that can meet a client's psychological need for security, a sense of belonging, and self-esteem.

a. _____

b. _____

c. _____

5. Place the phases of the human sexual response in the proper sequence.

_____ Plateau

_____ Resolution

_____ Orgasm

_____ Excitement

6. Match the term in the left column with its definition from the right column.

_____ sexuality   a. The belief that one is psychologically of the sex opposite to his or her anatomic gender

_____ sex roles   b. The human characteristic that refers to all aspects of being male or female, including feelings, attitudes, beliefs, and behavior

_____ gender identity   c. Having an equal or almost equal preference for partners of either sex

_____ sexual orientation   d. How one views oneself as male or female in relationship to others

_____ heterosexuality   e. Culturally determined patterns of behavior associated with being male and female

_____ homosexuality   f. Sexual activity between two members of the same sex

_____ bisexuality   g. Sexual activity between a man and a woman

_____ transsexuality   h. An individual's preference for expressing sexual feelings

7. Which activity is a health-promoting behavior?

a. Alcohol intake

b. Sleeping 5 hours a night

c. Breast self-examination

d. Walking

© 2011 Cengage Learning. All Rights Reserved. May not be scanned, copied or duplicated, or posted to a publicly accessible website, in whole or in part.

8. Which of the following terms describes an individual's perception of his or her own ability to perform a certain task?

    a. Empowerment

    b. Self-efficacy

    c. Self-concept

    d. Self-esteem

9. A client newly diagnosed with lung cancer states, "I have taken good care of myself and don't know how I am going to cope with this. What should I do?" Which response would best support this client's emotional and spiritual needs?

    a. "I will ask your prescribing practitioner to get a consult with the staff social worker."

    b. "Next time the hospital chaplain is here, I will ask him to stop by to see you."

    c. "Let me get your medications; you will feel better after you take them."

    d. "Tell me more about your situation. I have a few minutes; I can stay and talk awhile."

10. Which type of medication is associated with sexual dysfunction?

    a. Antihypertensives

    b. Antipyretics

    c. Antidiabetics

    d. Anticoagulants

11. Match the leading health indicators to the Healthy People 2010 objectives.

    _____   promoting healthy behaviors   a. Food production

    _____   promoting healthy and safe communities   b. Physical activity

    _____   improving personal and public health   c. Injury prevention

    _____   preventing and reducing diseases and disorders   d. Mental illness

12. Which disease process would be considered chronic?

    a. Pneumonia

    b. Poison ivy

    c. Diabetes

    d. Influenza

© 2011 Cengage Learning. All Rights Reserved. May not be scanned, copied or duplicated, or posted to a publicly accessible website, in whole or in part.

13. Disease prevention occurs on a continuum. Which is an example of *tertiary* prevention?

   a. A nurse conducts parenting classes at the local hospital.

   b. The local hospital offers blood pressure screening clinics once a month.

   c. A local health maintenance organization (HMO) offers stress management classes.

   d. A nurse works in a short-term rehabilitation facility assisting stroke clients to regain functional ability.

14. For a nurse to be an effective change agent when assisting clients to adopt a healthier lifestyle, which would a nurse incorporate into the care plan?

   a. A standard, unmodified teaching plan for all clients

   b. The client's individual beliefs and motivations for change

   c. Regular appointments for a check-up

   d. Enrolling the client in a wellness program

15. Which is an example of an intervention that empowers the client?

   a. Linking a breastfeeding mother with La Leche League International

   b. Arranging for the spouse of a fully functioning client to manage and administer the client's medication in the home environment

   c. Feeding a client when the client is able to feed himself or herself

   d. Planning a bathing and grooming schedule for a functioning client

16. A client says to the nurse, "I can manage this disease. I just need to learn more about it and what I can do to stay healthy." What does the nurse realize this client is demonstrating?

   a. Internal locus of control

   b. External locus of control

   c. Self-concept

   d. Self-image

17. A client tells the nurse that she gets an annual mammogram and does monthly breast self-examinations. In which type of activity is the client participating?

   a. Primary prevention

   b. Secondary prevention

   c. Tertiary prevention

   d. High-level wellness

© 2011 Cengage Learning. All Rights Reserved. May not be scanned, copied or duplicated, or posted to a publicly accessible website, in whole or in part.

18. The nurse is planning an educational session on sexuality for a group of adolescents. Which topic should be included in this session?

    a. Erectile dysfunction

    b. Use of lubricants

    c. Differentiation between "good" touching and "bad" touching

    d. Sexual abuse prevention

Critical Thinking

19. How does the clinical model of health differ from the health promotion model of health?

20. Discuss how individuals can become more responsible for their own health.

Activities

21. Identify a specific period of time in the evening to view a television show. During the show, count the number of commercials that appear. Identify the content of each commercial. Categorize the commercials as health promoting or non–health promoting. Examples of health promotion are exercise, diet, weight management, safety features on automobiles, and so forth. Examples of non–health promotion are fast food restaurants, alcohol consumption, other high-calorie foods, and so forth. Discuss how exposure to these types of commercials, both health promoting and non–health promoting, can influence the choices that Americans make.

22. Conduct an Internet search on the types of "alternative" medicine approaches available today. Focus on one specific alternative medicine approach. What is it primarily used for? What does it claim to help or prevent? Is there any scientific evidence to support the approach? Discuss the information learned.

23. The area of assessment that nurses have the most difficulty with is sexuality. In small groups, discuss why talking about sexuality with another person or client is difficult. What can be done to prepare in advance for a discussion about sexuality with a client?

© 2011 Cengage Learning. All Rights Reserved. May not be scanned, copied or duplicated, or posted to a publicly accessible website, in whole or in part.

Chapter 17 Family and Community Health

1. The following terms are related to community health nursing care. Match the terms with the description.

   _____ family   a. Basic unit of society

   _____ family roles   b. Roles that allow adaptation

   _____ family functions   c. Maintains family function

   _____ family structure   d. Behaviors expected of members

2. Which best describes the typical family form?

   a. Nuclear

   b. Blended

   c. Extended

   d. There is no typical family structure.

3. A combination of two divorced families through remarriage is termed a(n)

   a. extended family.

   b. blended family.

   c. dual-career family.

   d. compounded family.

4. Which question would a family nurse use to assess a family?

   a. How has your adult child returning home to live affected your relationship with your husband?

   b. How are your siblings integrated with your family?

   c. What problems are your children having in school?

   d. What support agencies does your family use?

© 2011 Cengage Learning. All Rights Reserved. May not be scanned, copied or duplicated, or posted to a publicly accessible website, in whole or in part.

5.   A healthy family is characterized by

   a.   teaching respect for others.

   b.   group communication.

   c.   parents acting as a team.

   d.   trust.

6.   A family lacking problem-solving skills and that is overinvolved is termed

   _____.

7.   A developmental task of middle-aged parents, according to McGoldrick and Carter, is to

   a.   incorporate new members into the family unit.

   b.   launch the children.

   c.   reinvest in couple identity.

   d.   accept the reality of death.

8.   Domestic violence occurs in

   a.   lower socioeconomic groups.

   b.   dysfunctional parent families.

   c.   all socioeconomic groups.

   d.   healthy families only.

9.   Victims of violence are primarily

   a.   children.

   b.   elderly.

   c.   spouses.

   d.   all of the above.

10.   Identify the true statement.

   a.   There is no link between childhood abuse and adult abuse.

   b.   Children suffer from family violence when they are direct victims.

   c.   Children who have been abused may think violence is normal behavior.

   d.   Violence between spouses is rare.

© 2011 Cengage Learning. All Rights Reserved. May not be scanned, copied or duplicated, or posted to a publicly accessible website, in whole or in part.

11. The mother of a 24-month-old infant talks about feeling "overwhelmed" and "out of control." The nurse learns that the mother has few social supports. What can the nurse suggest to this mother?

    a. Hotline for parents to talk with a helpful person

    b. Behavior management group

    c. Social worker visit

    d. Hiring a babysitter

12. A healthy community provides its residents with

    a. quality medical care.

    b. a safe environment.

    c. a place for growth.

    d. all of the above.

13. Settings for community health nurses include

    a. emergency departments.

    b. psychiatric units.

    c. primary care offices.

    d. hospitals.

14. Which nurse has the unique opportunity to detect indications of abuse?

    a. Acute care nurse

    b. Intensive care nurse

    c. Home care nurse

    d. Outpatient surgical nurse

15. The distribution and determinant of health and illness states in a population is defined as

    a. an aggregate.

    b. community statistics.

    c. epidemiology.

    d. prometrics.

© 2011 Cengage Learning. All Rights Reserved. May not be scanned, copied or duplicated, or posted to a publicly accessible website, in whole or in part.

16. The public health nurse specializes in community health nursing by

    a. focusing on illness prevention.

    b. staffing nursing clinics.

    c. working with individuals only.

    d. collecting statistical data.

17. A subgroup in a community, such as pregnant teenagers, is called a(n)

    _____.

18. Match each prevention on the left with the level it represents.

    _____ relocation of victims   a. Primary prevention

    _____ family therapy   b. Secondary prevention

    _____ behavior modification   c. Tertiary prevention

    _____ parenting classes

19. An example of a primary prevention would be

    a. use of infant car seat.

    b. testicular self-exam.

    c. counseling.

    d. rehabilitation.

20. An example of intimate partner violence would be

    a. date rape.

    b. overmedicating individuals.

    c. verbal abuse.

    d. social isolation.

Critical Thinking

21. Violence is a growing concern in health care. Explain what a nurse should do if a client appears to be a victim of violence.

22. A community health nurse is arriving at the scene of a tornado. Explain the role of the nurse in this situation.

© 2011 Cengage Learning. All Rights Reserved. May not be scanned, copied or duplicated, or posted to a publicly accessible website, in whole or in part.

Activities

23. Contact local agencies to ask community health nurses to come to the class and discuss the role they play in the health of the community in which they serve. What are the particular challenges they face? What are the opportunities? What successes have they had with the communities?

24. Access the Federal Emergency Management Agency Web site at http://www.fema.gov/areyouready. Click on the links under the "Are You Ready Guide" (left side of the screen). Discuss ways to individually prepare for natural and manmade disasters.

© 2011 Cengage Learning. All Rights Reserved. May not be scanned, copied or duplicated, or posted to a publicly accessible website, in whole or in part.

Chapter 18 The Life Cycle

1. During each developmental stage of the life cycle, developmental tasks must be achieved. Which phrase is the best example of the achievement of a developmental task?

   a. The normal physical development of a neonate occurs from newborn to preschool age.

   b. An adolescent forms relationships with members of the opposite sex.

   c. A woman experiences breast tenderness and engorgement during the first trimester of pregnancy.

   d. An elderly man loses interest in sex due to decreased levels of testosterone in the blood.

2. Which element influences a person's growth and development?

   a. Age

   b. Height

   c. Heredity

   d. Weight

3. Who developed a theory of moral development based on studies of women?

   a. Gilligan

   b. Kohlberg

   c. Piaget

   d. Sullivan

4. Who postulated that an individual's unconscious processes are a motivator of behavior?

   a. Freud

   b. Piaget

   c. Kohlberg

   d. Gilligan

© 2011 Cengage Learning. All Rights Reserved. May not be scanned, copied or duplicated, or posted to a publicly accessible website, in whole or in part.

5. According to Erikson's stages of psychosocial development, which stage of development would a person be in if the task to be achieved is to view one's life as meaningful and fulfilling?

   a. Identity vs. role diffusion

   b. Intimacy vs. isolation

   c. Generativity vs. stagnation

   d. Integrity vs. despair

6. Match Freud's psychosexual stage in the left column with its description from the right column.

   _____ oral   a. Emergence of sexual maturity and formation of relationships with potential sexual partners

   _____ anal   b. Management of anxiety by using mouth and tongue

   _____ phallic   c. Quiet stage during which sexual energy is repressed and sexual development lies dormant

   _____ latency   d. Awareness of sex and genitalia

   _____ genital   e. Control of muscles, especially those controlling urination and defecation

7. Identify the psychosocial changes of the older adult. (Select all that apply.)

   a. Satisfaction with life

   b. Empty nest syndrome

   c. Adjustment to infirmities

   d. Preparing for death

8. A major psychological task of neonates is to _____ with parents.

9. At which stage of Piaget's phases of cognitive development is the ability to see relationships and to do abstract thinking developed?

   a. Sensorimotor

   b. Preoperational

   c. Concrete operations

   d. Formal operations

© 2011 Cengage Learning. All Rights Reserved. May not be scanned, copied or duplicated, or posted to a publicly accessible website, in whole or in part.

10. At what age would you expect a child to form short, simple sentences?

   a. 1 year

   b. 18 months

   c. 2 years

   d. 3 years

11. Place the following stages of faith, according to Fowler, in the proper sequence.

   _____   Conjunctive faith

   _____   Universalizing faith

   _____   Intuitive-projective faith

   _____   Mythical-literal faith

   _____   Undifferentiated faith

   _____   Individuative-reflective faith

   _____   Synthetic-conventional faith

12. In which trimester of pregnancy is the fetus most susceptible to the effects of alcohol and other teratogenic substances?

   a. First

   b. Second

   c. Third

13. Which characteristic is an advantage of breast milk?

   a. Is easily digested

   b. Is higher in fat

   c. Has larger curds than cow's milk

   d. Is higher in carbohydrates

14. Which of the following is the leading cause of death in young children?

   a. Suicide

   b. Respiratory disease

   c. Sports injuries

   d. Accidents

© 2011 Cengage Learning. All Rights Reserved. May not be scanned, copied or duplicated, or posted to a publicly accessible website, in whole or in part.

15. When teaching a preadolescent female about menstrual periods, which of the following statements would be accurate to relate?

    a. The average age of menarche is 10 years old.

    b. The menstrual cycle becomes regular after about 6–12 months.

    c. Approximately 40% of American females experience premenstrual syndrome.

    d. During the first few menstrual cycles, females do not ovulate.

16. In which age group are individuals at the highest risk for suicide?

    a. Preadolescent

    b. Adolescent

    c. Young adult

    d. Middle adult

17. A 16-year-old male comes to the school nurse complaining of urethritis, purulent discharge, urinary frequency, and inflammation of the epididymis. Of which STD is this client demonstrating symptoms?

    a. Chlamydia

    b. Gonorrhea

    c. Genital warts

    d. Trichomoniasis

18. Which would be appropriate to teach a middle-aged adult regarding physiological changes?

    a. Explain to men that enlargement of the prostate gland is common.

    b. Encourage a balance of exercise/activity and rest and sleep.

    c. Teach about fall precaution measures.

    d. Teach about the need for adequate calcium intake.

19. Which would be the focus of a wellness program for middle-aged adults?

    a. Stress management

    b. Fall prevention

    c. Suicide prevention

    d. Increased socialization

© 2011 Cengage Learning. All Rights Reserved. May not be scanned, copied or duplicated, or posted to a publicly accessible website, in whole or in part.

20. Which statement is true of older adults?

    a. The majority are in nursing homes.

    b. There is no decline in IQ with advancing age.

    c. Most older adults suffer from debilitating illnesses.

    d. There are minimal visual changes associated with aging.

21. Which schedule is recommended for immunization of normal infants and children in the first year of life?

    a. Birth, 2 months, 6 months, 12 months

    b. 1 month, 3 months, 9 months

    c. Birth, 2 months, 6 months, 15 months

    d. Birth, 6 months, 24 months

Critical Thinking

22. Discuss the Centers for Disease Control and Prevention's Health Protection Goals for healthy people in every stage of life.

23. Discuss the recommended immunizations for the adult client.

Activities

24. Research your own history of immunizations. Contact your primary care prescribing practitioner, or talk with your parents to determine which immunizations you received and the date. At what ages were the immunizations provided? Have the recommended ages for the immunizations changed since you received them? Study the Recommended Adult Immunization Schedule and determine if all your immunizations are current. What immunizations are lacking? Why have they not been received? Discuss the impact of having immunizations current and up to date.

25. Invite a variety of children (with parents) of different ages to the classroom. Have items for play available and appropriate to each age represented. Spend time with each child, and identify developmental stages for the child's age. Talk with the parents as well to identify their developmental stages and levels. If time permits, prepare a presentation to discuss safety issues with those present. Ensure that the presentation addresses safety issues appropriate for all ages of those present.

© 2011 Cengage Learning. All Rights Reserved. May not be scanned, copied or duplicated, or posted to a publicly accessible website, in whole or in part.

Chapter 19 The Older Client

1. The process of stereotyping and discriminating against people because they are old defines

   _____.

2. Which is the greatest problem in the homebound elderly?

   a. Malnutrition

   b. Kidney stones

   c. Uncontrolled diabetes

   d. Loneliness

3. Contributing factors to erectile dysfunction in older men are

   a. anemia.

   b. diabetes.

   c. hypertension.

   d. medications.

   e. all of the above.

4. An expectation of the older adult in this stage of growth and development is to accept one's life as it is. Which action would facilitate this goal?

   a. Encourage the use of reminiscence.

   b. Assess for body image changes.

   c. Instruct about the benefits of proper nutrition and exercise.

   d. Encourage socialization.

5. The hearing loss associated with old age is called

   a. presbycusis.

   b. presbyopia.

   c. presbycardia.

   d. otitis media.

© 2011 Cengage Learning. All Rights Reserved. May not be scanned, copied or duplicated, or posted to a publicly accessible website, in whole or in part.

6. Match the pathological visual change experienced by the elderly in the left column with its description from the right column.

_____ macular degeneration   a. Opacity of the lens of the eye

_____ cataracts   b. Inability of the lens to accommodate for near vision

_____ glaucoma   c. Increased intraocular pressure

_____ presbyopia   d. Loss of central vision

7. Which physiological change associated with aging would support the need to teach a preoperative 78-year-old client deep breathing, coughing, and incentive spirometry exercises?

   a. Fewer functioning alveoli and decrease in the number of cilia

   b. Decrease in peristaltic activity

   c. Slowed transmission of nerve impulses

   d. The development of lentigo senilis

8. A 90-year-old client has visual deficit. All the following nursing interventions would enhance the client's lifestyle *except*

   a. large-print books.

   b. books on tape.

   c. color-coded stove dials.

   d. a TDD phone.

9. Aging is associated with altered functioning of the pancreas. Which would a nurse evaluate in order to assess this problem?

   a. Blood glucose level

   b. Blood urea nitrogen level

   c. Bowel sounds

   d. Blood potassium level

10. Which normal genitourinary symptom is associated with the normal aging process?

   a. Nocturia

   b. Pain with urination

   c. Bladder infections

   d. Kidney stones

© 2011 Cengage Learning. All Rights Reserved. May not be scanned, copied or duplicated, or posted to a publicly accessible website, in whole or in part.

11.   An elderly client has kyphosis and osteoporosis. The nurse realizes that these health issues are most likely because of

   a.   inactivity.

   b.   malnutrition.

   c.   smoking.

   d.   estrogen loss.

12.   Which statement is true regarding wound healing in the elderly? Wounds heal

   a.   at the same rate as in middle-aged adults.

   b.   faster than in middle-aged adults.

   c.   slower than in middle-aged adults.

   d.   at a rate that depends on the client's age.

13.   Which strategy would be appropriate to teach an elderly client regarding skin care?

   a.   Avoid tub baths.

   b.   Use tepid water during baths.

   c.   Rub the skin briskly while drying the skin.

   d.   Use alcohol to soothe itchy, dry skin areas.

14.   An 82-year-old client is admitted with pneumonia. Currently the client has a low-grade fever with dehydration. She is disoriented, mumbles incoherently, cannot feed herself, and sees bugs crawling in her room. Her family states that the client was oriented and alert at home. What is this client most likely experiencing?

   a.   Acute confusion

   b.   Dementia

   c.   An episode of depression

   d.   A personality disorder

15.   What is the greatest risk of developing adverse drug reactions in the elderly?

   a.   Expensive drug costs

   b.   Noncompliance

   c.   Polypharmacy

   d.   Medication errors

© 2011 Cengage Learning. All Rights Reserved. May not be scanned, copied or duplicated, or posted to a publicly accessible website, in whole or in part.

16. Match the age-related change in the left column with its impact on drug therapy from the right column.

_____	less total body fluid	a.	Difficulty absorbing usual intramuscular adult dose at a single injection site
_____	increased adipose tissue	b.	Higher level of water-soluble drugs
_____	reduced liver size and decreased hepatic metabolism	c.	Greater accumulation of fat-soluble drugs
_____	reduced glomerular filtration rate and decreased number of nephrons	d.	Slower metabolism and longer half-life of some drugs
_____	drier oral mucosa	e.	Prolonged melting times for suppositories
_____	less muscle mass	f.	Difficulty swallowing tablets and capsules
_____	reduced circulation to lower bowel and vagina	g.	Slower elimination of some drugs

17. When taking a medication history of an elderly client, which should be assessed in addition to the client's prescription drugs?

    a. Potential interactions with foods

    b. Use of over-the-counter medications

    c. How medications are obtained

    d. All of the above

18. Which type of elder abuse is imposed social isolation?

    a. Psychological abuse

    b. Physical abuse

    c. Neglect

    d. Exploitation

19. List three age-related factors that contribute to falls.

    a. _____

    b. _____

    c. _____

© 2011 Cengage Learning. All Rights Reserved. May not be scanned, copied or duplicated, or posted to a publicly accessible website, in whole or in part.

20.   Which intervention would promote the safety of an elderly client admitted to a long-term care facility?

    a.   Teach about correct medication administration.

    b.   Orient to surroundings.

    c.   Provide large-print materials to read.

    d.   Help to focus the client on abilities instead of limitations.

Critical Thinking

21.   Discuss ways to ensure medication adherence in the elderly client.

22.   An elderly client tells the nurse that she cannot afford her medications because her son needs money to pay off bills. Discuss what this situation implies and what the nurse can do to help the client.

Activities

23.   Identify adult day care or senior centers in the community. Schedule time to either visit the facilities or invite participants to come to the classroom to discuss the activities provided through the facilities. Ask the participants what attending these programs does to enhance their socialization.

24.   Contact the community Center for Aging or Adult Protective Services program. Invite the coordinator of either program to come to the class to discuss the programs and services offered to the elderly.

25.   Research magazines, newspapers, or other print media to determine how the media portrays the elderly. Share the information obtained with the class.

© 2011 Cengage Learning. All Rights Reserved. May not be scanned, copied or duplicated, or posted to a publicly accessible website, in whole or in part.

Chapter 20 Cultural Diversity

1. Match the term in the left column with its definition from the right column.

   _____ culture

   a. The dynamic and integrated structures of knowledge, beliefs, behaviors, ideas, values, habits, customs, languages, symbols, rituals, ceremonies, and practices unique to a particular group of people

   _____ ethnicity

   b. A group that constitutes less than the majority of the population

   _____ race

   c. The group whose values prevail in a society

   _____ stereotyping

   d. A grouping of people based on biological similarities

   _____ dominant culture

   e. Labeling people based on cultural preconceptions

   _____ minority group

   f. A cultural group's perception of itself

2. Which is the largest minority group in the United States?

   a. European American

   b. Hispanic

   c. African American

   d. American Indian

3. There are six organizing factors nurses must consider when delivering culturally competent care: space, orientation to time, social organization, environmental control, biological variations, and

   _____.

4. Match the cultural group in the left column with the disorder most likely to affect the group from the right column.

   _____ African American   a. Heart disease

   _____ Asian American   b. Glaucoma

   _____ European American   c. Lactose intolerance

   _____ Native American, Eskimo   d. Sickle cell anemia

© 2011 Cengage Learning. All Rights Reserved. May not be scanned, copied or duplicated, or posted to a publicly accessible website, in whole or in part.

5. In which cultural group is eye contact considered a sign of disrespect?

   a. European American

   b. Native American

   c. Hispanic American

   d. African American

6. Which communication technique would *not* be culturally appropriate?

   a. Active listening

   b. Silence

   c. Slow speech

   d. Loud and clear speech

7. In which culture does the family assume greater importance than the individual?

   a. Gay

   b. Middle-class European American

   c. Hispanic

   d. Upper-class European American

8. Which cultural characteristic is defined as cultural change occurring slowly in response to group needs?

   a. Learned and taught

   b. Shared

   c. Social in nature

   d. Dynamic and adaptive

9. Which best explains the purpose of the U.S. government WIC program?

   a. It provides individuals diagnosed with AIDS without income with supplemental income.

   b. It provides the homeless with shelter.

   c. It provides pregnant and breastfeeding mothers with supplemental food and other health services.

   d. It provides homeless children with food, shelter, and clothing.

© 2011 Cengage Learning. All Rights Reserved. May not be scanned, copied or duplicated, or posted to a publicly accessible website, in whole or in part.

10. Which health problem would you expect to find among the homeless?

    a. Stroke

    b. Respiratory diseases

    c. Arthritis

    d. Keloid formation

11. Which cultural group avoids physical closeness?

    a. African American

    b. Asian American

    c. Hispanic American

    d. Native American

12. Match the cultural group in the left column with its traditional healer from the right column.

    _____   African American   a. Herbalist

    _____   Asian American   b. Shaman

    _____   European American   c. *Curandero*

    _____   Hispanic American   d. "Community Mother"

    _____   Native American   e. Prescribing practitioner

13. In which cultural group would antihypertensives be administered in higher doses?

    a. African American

    b. Asian American

    c. Native American

    d. European American

14. Which approach is essential to the delivery of culturally sensitive care?

    a. Technical competence

    b. Detailed knowledge of the client's culture

    c. A nonjudgmental attitude

    d. Fluency in the client's native language

© 2011 Cengage Learning. All Rights Reserved. May not be scanned, copied or duplicated, or posted to a publicly accessible website, in whole or in part.

15. The concept that individuals are absorbed into the predominant group is called

  a. cultural relativity.

  b. cultural stereotyping.

  c. culturally sensitive interactions.

  d. cultural assimilation.

16. A client is admitted to the hospital and tells the nurse that he is married but has no children. The nurse would identify this family structure as

  a. incipient.

  b. nuclear.

  c. attenuated.

  d. blended.

17. In which cultural group will there be less respect for authority figures?

  a. Asian

  b. Upper-class Euro-American

  c. Hispanic

  d. Middle-class Euro-American

18. While assessing a client from a different culture, the nurse notes that the client is wearing a black stone on a chain as a necklace. The cultural group that uses this stone as a healing practice is

  a. African American.

  b. Hispanic American.

  c. Asian American.

  d. Native American.

19. In which cultural group is the development of diabetes least likely to occur?

  a. African American

  b. Hispanic American

  c. Asian American

  d. Native American

© 2011 Cengage Learning. All Rights Reserved. May not be scanned, copied or duplicated, or posted to a publicly accessible website, in whole or in part.

Critical Thinking

20.   Describe the concept of ethnocentrism and how it impacts the way other cultures are respected.

21.   Explain why the treatment for tuberculosis might be a challenge in a person of African, Asian, or Native American descent.

Activities

22.   Identify the cultural group for every member of the class. What information provided in the chapter regarding family structure, communication, space, time orientation, environmental control, and biological variations does each class member identify within themselves? Discuss the information in small groups.

23.   Contact local organizations for information about the area's homeless community. Invite community leaders who are active in the homeless community to the classroom to discuss the challenges and opportunities with the community. What programs are provided for these citizens? What health care programs are available to them? What is the community doing to reduce or eliminate homelessness?

24.   Depending on availability, invite a person of a different culture to the class to discuss the difference in health care between his or her native country and the United States. What can be done to improve the health care of the culture? What challenges does he or she experience when accessing health care in the United States?

© 2011 Cengage Learning. All Rights Reserved. May not be scanned, copied or duplicated, or posted to a publicly accessible website, in whole or in part.

Chapter 21   Client Education

1. Which statement indicates that a client is ready to learn about diabetes? The client states:

   a. "I will go to the diabetes class tomorrow."

   b. "Tell my wife about my diabetes. She is better at remembering that sort of stuff."

   c. "My doctor tells me I should learn more about the foods I should or should not eat."

   d. "Show me how to inject myself with insulin."

2. A client received learning materials about how to care for himself at home after surgery. Which request would best determine that the client understands how to care for an incision?

   a. You ask him if he has read the booklet.

   b. You ask him to explain how to care for his incision.

   c. You show him how to cleanse the incision and apply a dressing.

   d. You ask his wife if the client understands how to care for his incision.

3. A 75-year-old client has just been taught how to self-administer eye drops. Which activity would validate that learning has occurred?

   a. Discussion

   b. Continued observation

   c. Listening and viewing audiovisual material

   d. Return demonstration

4. Prior to teaching a 35-year-old client how to test his blood glucose, what should the nurse assess?

   a. Knowledge about diabetes

   b. Ability to use a glucometer

   c. Readiness to learn

   d. Reading level

© 2011 Cengage Learning. All Rights Reserved. May not be scanned, copied or duplicated, or posted to a publicly accessible website, in whole or in part.

5. Organizing content from the simple to the complex makes the learning process proceed in a user-friendly direction. Which learning theorist would subscribe to this principle?

   a. Ivan Pavlov

   b. John Dewey

   c. Jerome Bruner

   d. Robert Gagne

6. A client who needs to learn how to self-administer insulin tells the nurse that he learns best "by doing." This is an example of a _____ learning style.

7. Match the age group in the left column with the appropriate teaching strategy for that age group from the right column.

   _____ children   a. Use play and imitation.

   _____ adolescents   b. Use silence to allow time to process information.

   _____ middle-aged adults   c. Identify and build on positive qualities.

   _____ older adults   d. Prepare print-based material at an appropriate reading skill level.

8. A client diagnosed with hypertension is referred for diet and medication counseling. Which phase of care does the referral reflect?

   a. Primary

   b. Secondary

   c. Tertiary

   d. Restorative

9. A nurse considers the who, what, when, and where of client teaching in which phase of the teaching-learning process?

   a. Assessment

   b. Identification of learning needs

   c. Planning

   d. Implementation

© 2011 Cengage Learning. All Rights Reserved. May not be scanned, copied or duplicated, or posted to a publicly accessible website, in whole or in part.

10. A client who was admitted for hypertensive crisis because he did not take his medications will be discharged in a few days. Which assessment is a priority when determining his discharge planning needs?

   a. His ability to purchase his medications

   b. The cleanliness of his home

   c. The availability of someone to help with his care

   d. The availability of a hypertension education group in his immediate area

11. A client admitted with generalized anxiety order has the goal of "I will develop and use coping skills to manage my anxiety." Which statement supports that the client has met the goal?

   a. "I can cope with my stressors."

   b. "My anxiety level is manageable at a level of 2 on a scale of 1 to 5."

   c. "I know what stress management techniques I need to learn in order to cope."

   d. "My nurse will tell me when I need to calm down."

12. Which client is in need of learning?

   a. A client newly diagnosed with diabetes

   b. A client experiencing new onset of back pain

   c. A client having an outpatient surgical procedure for breast biopsy

   d. All of the above

13. A client has the teaching outcome of "Client will state signs and symptoms of gastrointestinal bleeding and report them to the nurse or prescribing practitioner." Which form of documentation reflects that the standard has been met for this client's teaching?

   a. Client was taught the information and seemed to understand it.

   b. Client was read the materials about the signs and symptoms of GI bleeding and said he would take the information home with him.

   c. Client was asked about the signs and symptoms of gastrointestinal bleeding, questions were answered, and he seemed satisfied with the information.

   d. Client was given written information about the signs and symptoms of gastrointestinal bleeding. It was reviewed with him. He gave correct responses to follow-up questions.

© 2011 Cengage Learning. All Rights Reserved. May not be scanned, copied or duplicated, or posted to a publicly accessible website, in whole or in part.

14. How can the nurse determine the priority learning needs of a client?

    a. Review the list of client learning outcomes.

    b. Conduct a comprehensive learning needs assessment.

    c. Identify the actual and potential learning needs and address the actual needs first.

    d. Ask the client if there are any questions you can answer.

15. Which client is demonstrating a high readiness to learn?

    a. A client crying quietly after the prescribing practitioner has left the room

    b. A client waiting for pain medication after hip replacement surgery

    c. A client sitting quietly in the room, with no complaints of pain, waiting for the lunch tray

    d. A client recovering from 2 days of nausea and vomiting who is receiving intravenous fluids and electrolyte replacements for dehydration

16. Which concept is linked to motivation to learn?

    a. Self-efficacy

    b. Self-esteem

    c. Self-care

    d. Learning ability

17. Which learning goal is stated correctly?

    a. Client will state the side effects of digoxin.

    b. By discharge, the client will be able to select foods that contain vitamin K and state which foods are to be avoided.

    c. By the surgical date, the client will have read the preoperative instructions.

    d. Within 1 week, the client will learn how to use a walker.

18. Which organization mandates client teaching?

    a. All state boards of nursing

    b. NLN

    c. Joint Commission

    d. American Nurses Association

© 2011 Cengage Learning. All Rights Reserved. May not be scanned, copied or duplicated, or posted to a publicly accessible website, in whole or in part.

19. A peak in the effectiveness of teaching and depth of learning is called a

_____.

20. It is important for nurses to know the reading and comprehension abilities of clients before using written materials in the teaching process. Which percentage of the U.S. population has limited health literacy?

    a. 50%

    b. 25%

    c. 33%

    d. 20%

Critical Thinking

21. Discuss the different categories of client education.

22. Explain the role of repetition in learning.

Activities

23. Create a teaching topic plan for clients with the following health problems:

    a. Insufficient protein intake

    b. Nerve damage due to spinal cord compression

    c. Activity intolerance due to cardiac disease

    Divide the class into small groups, and discuss the topics that would be appropriate for each health problem.

24. Using the Internet, research a variety of client educational Web sites available by typing "patient education" on the Google search page at http://www.google.com. Access the Merck Medicus client education Web site at http://www.merckmedicus.com/pp/us/hcp/templates/tier2/patientEdu.jsp, and review the latest client handouts.

© 2011 Cengage Learning. All Rights Reserved. May not be scanned, copied or duplicated, or posted to a publicly accessible website, in whole or in part.

Chapter 22 Self-Concept

1. Match the term in the left column with its definition from the right column.

    _____ identity

    _____ body image

    _____ role

    _____ self-esteem

    a. What an individual thinks he or she looks like

    b. Set of expected behaviors determined by family, culture, and society

    c. A person's sense of self-worth

    d. The set of characteristics a person is recognized by

2. Within which life stage does the self-concept develop and change?

    a. Childhood

    b. Adolescence

    c. Adulthood

    d. All of the above

3. Which behavior might suggest a nursing diagnosis of altered self-concept?

    a. Lack of eye contact

    b. Hesitant speech

    c. Unusual dependence

    d. All of the above

4. A nurse has school, family, and work demands and is having difficulty prioritizing tasks. Which type of role conflict does this situation describe?

    a. Interrole conflict

    b. Interpersonal role conflict

    c. Role overload

    d. Person-role conflict

© 2011 Cengage Learning. All Rights Reserved. May not be scanned, copied or duplicated, or posted to a publicly accessible website, in whole or in part.

5. A nurse asks a client the following question during an interview: "What are your strengths and weaknesses?" Which aspect of the self-concept does this question assess?

   a. Body image

   b. Identity

   c. Role

   d. Self-esteem

6. A client experiencing symptoms of early menopause tells the nurse that she feels "old." Which intervention would best assist this client?

   a. Tell the client that old people are in their 80s.

   b. Acknowledge the client's concerns about feeling old.

   c. Discuss hormone replacement therapy with the client.

   d. Emphasize the benefits of early menopause.

7. A 59-year-old client admitted with a gastrointestinal bleed becomes angry when interrupted during a telephone call and tells the nurse that he does not need medication because there is "nothing wrong" with him. Which nursing diagnosis would be appropriate for this client?

   a. *Alteration in defense mechanisms*

   b. *Self-concept disturbance*

   c. *Hopelessness*

   d. *Social isolation*

8. A 16-year old-female admitted with the diagnosis of anorexia refuses to eat her meal and tells the nurse that she is "too fat." Which nursing diagnosis would be most appropriate for this client?

   a. *Situational low self-esteem*

   b. *Anxiety*

   c. *Body image disturbance*

   d. *Self-esteem disturbance*

© 2011 Cengage Learning. All Rights Reserved. May not be scanned, copied or duplicated, or posted to a publicly accessible website, in whole or in part.

9. Which nursing intervention is directed at minimizing stress associated with illness?

    a. Verbally instructing the client's spouse about effects and side effects of medications

    b. Allowing the client to make decisions about timing of care activities

    c. Directing the client to ask the prescribing practitioner about postoperative care during hospitalization

    d. Asking the client how he or she has coped with past illnesses

10. A client on bedrest tells the nurse that she needs to use the commode but feels uncomfortable because she does not have privacy. Which illness stressor is this client experiencing?

    a. Threat to physical safety

    b. Threat to psychological integrity

    c. Inability to exert control

    d. Unmet biological needs

11. Which of the following goals would be appropriate for a client experiencing *Situational low self-esteem?*

    a. The client will experience self-esteem.

    b. The client will state his positive attributes.

    c. The nurse will support the client's weaknesses.

    d. The nurse will facilitate the client's growth.

12. The nurse is planning the care of a client with a low self-concept. Which intervention would support therapeutic interactions with this client?

    a. Engage in active listening.

    b. Minimize interactions.

    c. Perform basic care activities for the client.

    d. Take away the client's defense processes.

© 2011 Cengage Learning. All Rights Reserved. May not be scanned, copied or duplicated, or posted to a publicly accessible website, in whole or in part.

13. A nurse is well groomed with erect posture and clear articulation when speaking. This nurse has positive relationships, is self-directed, and takes care of herself. This nurse is demonstrating

    a. high self-esteem.

    b. role satisfaction.

    c. personal identity.

    d. low self-esteem.

14. In which life stage would an individual's self-concept be most influenced by feedback from significant others?

    a. Childhood

    b. Adolescence

    c. Adulthood

    d. All of the above

15. Which statement is true about self-concept?

    a. Self-concept is an individual's perception of self.

    b. Self-concept is the perception of others about an individual.

    c. Self-concept is the reflection of an individual's achievements.

    d. Self-concept is derived from the expectations of others for an individual.

16. The nurse observes a parent ask a child, "Why can't you behave like your brother does?" What kind of response does this statement promote?

    a. Positive self-concept

    b. Role confusion

    c. Person-role conflict

    d. Negative self-concept

17. A client tells the nurse that she has to go home soon because her family "needs her." Which indicator of self-esteem is the client demonstrating?

    a. Behavior

    b. Decision making

    c. Self-care

    d. Measure of worth

© 2011 Cengage Learning. All Rights Reserved. May not be scanned, copied or duplicated, or posted to a publicly accessible website, in whole or in part.

Critical Thinking

18.   Discuss how a nurse can develop personal low self-esteem.

19.   Explain how a nurse can support a client's psychosocial need for self-esteem.

Activities

20.   Analyze your own self-concept. To do this, begin by defining personal identity: name, gender, ethnic identity, family status, and various roles. Next, identify body image. How do you see yourself? What do others say about you? Then, utilizing Table 22-4, assess your own level of self-esteem by using the indicators provided. Last, identify how you believe you are performing the roles identified in Step 1 of the process. Once this process is complete, divide the class into small groups and discuss the information gathered.

21.   Schedule a time when class members can attend a preschool or day care center for children. Observe the preschool/day care attendants' behaviors with the children. Do the attendants support the children's development of a positive self-concept? What behaviors are demonstrated? If the attendants do not support a positive self-concept, what behaviors are demonstrated?

22.   If possible, invite a psychologist or psychiatrist to the class to discuss the impact of self-concept on the development of psychological problems. Prepare in advance by having a list of questions or possible scenarios to present to the mental health professional(s).

© 2011 Cengage Learning. All Rights Reserved. May not be scanned, copied or duplicated, or posted to a publicly accessible website, in whole or in part.

Chapter 23 Stress, Anxiety, Adaptation, and Change

1. Match the term in the left column with its definition from the right column.

   _____ stress

   _____ stressor

   _____ anxiety

   _____ adaptation

   _____ homeostasis

   _____ maladaptation

   _____ eustress

   _____ distress

   a. The body's reaction to any stimulus

   b. The ineffective response to stressors

   c. Any situation, event, or agent that threatens a person's security

   d. The process whereby a person adjusts to stressors

   e. Ineffective coping with stressors

   f. The type of stress that results in positive outcomes

   g. A subjective response to a threat to a person's well-being

   h. A steady state balancing physiological, psychological, sociocultural, intellectual, and spiritual needs

2. Which type of stressor is a hot, crowded, noisy subway?

   a. Physiological

   b. Psychological

   c. Environmental

   d. Sociocultural

3. A client tells the nurse that every time she thinks about her upcoming breast cancer surgery, her heart "starts racing." Which stage of the general adaptation syndrome response is the client describing?

   a. Stage I: alarm

   b. Stage II: resistance

   c. Stage III: exhaustion

   d. Stage I: autonomic nervous system response

© 2011 Cengage Learning. All Rights Reserved. May not be scanned, copied or duplicated, or posted to a publicly accessible website, in whole or in part.

4. Which is a cognitive manifestation of stress?

   a. Impaired judgment

   b. Headache

   c. Insomnia

   d. Social isolation

5. A client has just returned from abdominal surgery. Which of the body's physiological stress responses will he or she experience?

   a. Decreased urinary output

   b. Increased urinary output

   c. No change in output

   d. Inability to produce urine

6. A client tells the nurse that he is having trouble sleeping, cannot concentrate, argues with his wife, and is bored since retiring 1 month ago. Which type of crisis is the client demonstrating?

   a. Maturational

   b. Situational

   c. Adventitious

   d. Diabetic

7. Which is an appropriate nursing intervention for a client whose anxiety level is severe?

   a. Discuss medication side effects and dosing instructions.

   b. Assist the client in linking the stressor to the anxiety response.

   c. Invite the client to join a group on diet management.

   d. Use broad opening statements; allow the client an opportunity to discuss concerns.

8. The theorist who proposed that the change process occurs in the three stages of unfreezing, moving, and refreezing is

   a. Freud.

   b. Lippitt.

   c. Lewin.

   d. Nelson.

© 2011 Cengage Learning. All Rights Reserved. May not be scanned, copied or duplicated, or posted to a publicly accessible website, in whole or in part.

9.   Match the defense mechanism in the left column with an example of it from the right column.

_____   denial   a.   A nurse comes to work after an argument with her husband and becomes angry with the nurse's aide.

_____   displacement   b.   A workaholic mother brings a gift home every day to her child.

_____   rationalization c.   A client blames his wife for misplacing items when he cannot remember where he put things.

_____   regression   d.   A student nurse puts his children out of his mind while he is studying for an examination.

_____   suppression   e.   A client says he can't follow the prescribed diet because his wife doesn't know how to cook the proper foods.

_____   repression   f.   A client with cirrhosis continues to heavily drink alcohol.

_____   projection   g.   A 54-year-old client with bone cancer refuses to feed himself during hospitalization.

_____   reaction formation h.   A client is unaware of her sexual abuse history.

10.   When a client benefits from the sick role by gaining attention and sympathy, this is called a

_____.

11.   Which statement describes the relationship of stress to the body's immune functioning?

a.   Long-term stress enhances immune functioning.

b.   Short-term stress speeds up the healing process.

c.   There is no relationship between stress and the immune system.

d.   Long-term stress speeds up the healing process.

12.   A client is seen in the emergency department with a fractured arm. This client has experienced several losses over the last 6 months and tells the nurse that she keeps having accidents and "can't stop them." Which nursing diagnosis would be appropriate for this client?

a.   *Ineffective denial*

b.   *Powerlessness*

c.   *Ineffective coping*

d.   *Depression*

© 2011 Cengage Learning. All Rights Reserved. May not be scanned, copied or duplicated, or posted to a publicly accessible website, in whole or in part.

13. Which phrase explains the benefits of catharsis as a therapeutic intervention for purposes of anxiety management?

    a. Once a feeling is described, it is real and can be dealt with.

    b. It reduces the tension in muscles.

    c. It clarifies the message of the sender for the receiver.

    d. It allows the nurse to offer an opinion on the client's experience.

14. One of the beneficial effects of exercise in managing stress is the stimulation of the production of endorphins. Which best describes endorphins? Endorphins are

    a. a group of naturally occurring, chemically related, long-chain hydroxy fatty acids that stimulate the contractility of smooth muscles.

    b. a group of opiate-like substances produced naturally by the brain that raise the body's pain threshold.

    c. a group of high-molecular-weight kininogens that increase the permeability of capillaries.

    d. intermediate products in the synthesis of norepinephrine, a neurotransmitter.

15. Which stress management strategy would be helpful for a client who is having difficulty falling asleep?

    a. Progressive muscle relaxation

    b. Exercise

    c. Guided imagery

    d. Aromatherapy

16. Match the stress management technique in the left column with its definition from the right column.

    _____ progressive muscle relaxation   a. The client tenses and releases muscle groups throughout the body, paying attention to sensations of tension and relaxation.

    _____ guided imagery   b. The client's perception and interpretations are altered by changing of the client's thoughts.

    _____ cognitive reframing   c. A client is guided through a pleasant scene, using all the senses, in order to become fully relaxed.

17. Which assessment would not be useful when evaluating the effectiveness of anxiety reduction strategies?

    a. Vital signs measurement

    b. Cognition

    c. Motor movement

    d. Oxygen saturation

© 2011 Cengage Learning. All Rights Reserved. May not be scanned, copied or duplicated, or posted to a publicly accessible website, in whole or in part.

18. A nurse is overstressed. Which product should this nurse avoid?

   a. Alcohol

   b. Tobacco

   c. Caffeine

   d. All of the above

19. Which action is a characteristic of hardiness?

   a. Challenge

   b. Surrender

   c. Critical thinking

   d. Delegation

20. Which hormone is *not* involved in the biological changes associated with the fight-or-flight responses?

   a. Adrenalin

   b. Thyroid hormone

   c. Norepinephrine

   d. Glucocorticoids

Critical Thinking

21. Explain how a mild level of anxiety can promote cognition whereas severe anxiety can hinder cognition.

22. Discuss why some people resist change.

© 2011 Cengage Learning. All Rights Reserved. May not be scanned, copied or duplicated, or posted to a publicly accessible website, in whole or in part.

Activities

23. The current health care industry is under scrutiny. Discuss ways in which changing the current health care environment could produce resistance by health care providers and clients.

24. Break into small groups, and discuss the methods you use to combat stress.

25. Invite a stress management counselor to the class. Ask the counselor to discuss techniques to reduce stress. Find out which ones are the most successful and why.

26. Locate a guided imagery CD, and play the CD in class. Darken the lights, have class members assume comfortable positions, and participate in the instructions on the CD. If you are unable to locate a guided imagery CD, find a progressive muscle relaxation CD and follow the same process.

© 2011 Cengage Learning. All Rights Reserved. May not be scanned, copied or duplicated, or posted to a publicly accessible website, in whole or in part.

Chapter 24 Spirituality

1. Define spirituality.

   _____

   _____

   _____

2. Spirituality consists of

   a. religious beliefs.

   b. formal ritual practices.

   c. a set of beliefs held by a group.

   d. an individual set of beliefs.

3. Nursing actions that would meet clients' spiritual needs include

   a. choosing clients with the nurse's same religious affiliation.

   b. telling the clients you are praying for them.

   c. accepting the religious philosophy a client acts upon through an affirming presence.

   d. writing a pastoral care referral.

4. A goal of holistic nursing is to

   a. connect with the self.

   b. pray with others and a higher power.

   c. promote spiritual well-being.

   d. offer reassurance that problems have meaning and resolution is possible.

5. According to research, clients most appreciate spiritual discussions when

   a. dealing with a loss.

   b. being examined by the prescribing practitioner.

   c. preparing for surgery.

   d. being discharged.

© 2011 Cengage Learning. All Rights Reserved. May not be scanned, copied or duplicated, or posted to a publicly accessible website, in whole or in part.

6. Match a or b to the terms in the right column.

    _____ universal   a. Religion

    _____ denominations   b. Spirituality

    _____ private

    _____ public

    _____ spontaneous

    _____ ritualistic

7. Choose which is an indicator of a client's and his family's spiritual focus.

    a. There are religious artifacts in the home.

    b. The family says grace before every meal.

    c. Spiritual messages are displayed in the environment.

    d. All of the above indicate spiritual focus.

8. The therapeutic presence of the nurse during a crisis allows the client to establish a sense of _____ and rapport, which is essential for successful spiritual care.

9. Spiritual distress is defined as _____.

10. Spirituality has been shown to be beneficial to clients' health by _____. (Select all that apply.)

    a. reducing stress

    b. decreasing blood pressure

    c. improving sleep patterns

    d. decreasing substance abuse

11. A client tells the nurse that he feels most at peace when he spends time outdoors. Which characteristic of spirituality is this client describing?

    a. Relationship with self

    b. Relationship with others

    c. Harmony with nature

    d. Relationship with a higher power

© 2011 Cengage Learning. All Rights Reserved. May not be scanned, copied or duplicated, or posted to a publicly accessible website, in whole or in part.

12.   A client of the religion of Islam has died. What should the nurse do to assist this client and the family?

    a.   Provide water and towels so the family can wash the body.

    b.   Provide information about autopsy.

    c.   Observe the family cross the arms of the deceased client.

    d.   Provide oil to anoint the body of the deceased client.

13.   Match the world religion with the health care belief.

    _____   Seventh Day Adventist   a.   Some believe in divine healing.

    _____   Baptist   b.   Anoint with oil and pray for those who are ill.

    _____   Buddhist   c.   Illness is negative karma.

    _____   Roman Catholic   d.   Abortion is prohibited.

14.   Match the following spiritual assessment concepts and questions.

    _____   meaning and purpose   a.   What brings you peace?

    _____   inner strengths   b.   How hopeful are you about your condition improving?

    _____   interconnectedness   c.   Can you get help when you need it?

15.   A client asks the nurse why "cancer happened to me." The nurse's reaction should focus on

    a.   suggesting a spiritual advisor.

    b.   giving the client control of his or her medication regime.

    c.   explaining his or her experiences and reactions to crisis.

    d.   encouraging the client to explore this with significant others.

16.   List five factors associated with spiritual distress.

    a.   _____

    b.   _____

    c.   _____

    d.   _____

    e.   _____

© 2011 Cengage Learning. All Rights Reserved. May not be scanned, copied or duplicated, or posted to a publicly accessible website, in whole or in part.

17. Which of the following would place a client at risk for spiritual distress?

    a. Anxiety

    b. Death of a loved one

    c. Pain

    d. Substance abuse

18. _____, a form of meditation in which the focus is on the present moment, is one way to heighten an appreciation of the spiritual aspects of one's life.

19. The Joint Commission requires that clients be asked if they would like to

    a. pray.

    b. meet with their spiritual leader or advisor.

    c. learn relaxation techniques.

    d. attend church services.

20. Spiritual care is a component of

    a. holistic care.

    b. cultural care.

    c. religious affiliations.

21. List three primary nursing diagnoses related to spirituality.

    a. _____

    b. _____

    c. _____

Critical Thinking

22. A client tells the nurse that he does not "believe in God." How can the nurse support this client spiritually?

23. Compare faith with hope.

© 2011 Cengage Learning. All Rights Reserved. May not be scanned, copied or duplicated, or posted to a publicly accessible website, in whole or in part.

Activities

24. Divide the class into small groups, and discuss each person's individual religion or spirituality preferences. Identify specific rituals or activities that are followed. What is the significance of these rituals or activities?

25. Invite different denominations of clergy, pastors, and other religious leaders to the classroom. Conduct a panel discussion that focuses on their role in helping members of their denomination with health issues, crises, and death. Ask the panel if there are any specific rituals that are conducted within their denomination and what the significance of each ritual is.

26. Explore personal responses to health issues or health crises. What did you do to support your own spiritual needs? To whom did you turn for assistance and help? What was the most important thing that brought you through the crisis or health issue? Discuss the personal introspections in small groups.

© 2011 Cengage Learning. All Rights Reserved. May not be scanned, copied or duplicated, or posted to a publicly accessible website, in whole or in part.

Chapter 25 Loss and Grief

1. Match the term in the left column with its definition from the right column.

    _____ actual loss

    a. Loss of a body part or body function

    _____ perceived loss

    b. Loss of an aspect of self that is not physical; for example, loss of humor

    _____ physical loss

    c. The period of grief following the death of a loved one

    _____ psychological loss

    d. An adaptive process related to loss

    _____ grief

    e. A series of intense physical and psychological responses that occur following a loss

    _____ mourning

    f. Loss felt by an individual but not tangible to others

    _____ bereavement

    g. Death of a loved one; theft of an object

2. All of these religious traditions support organ donation except _____. (Select all that apply.)

    a. Catholicism

    b. Judaism

    c. Christian Science

    d. Protestantism

    e. Hinduism

    f. Islam

3. A client's husband is troubled by his wife's illness of ovarian and uterine cancer. The client had been previously healthy and the husband wanted to have more children. The husband demonstrates anxious behavior when the nurse comes into the room. Which of the following identifies the losses this couple is experiencing?

    a. Loss of good health, goals, bodily function, and self-concept as a whole

    b. Loss of role relationship, body parts, hope, and job

    c. Loss of a significant other, self-concept, body parts, and support

    d. Loss of self-esteem, health, and support

© 2011 Cengage Learning. All Rights Reserved. May not be scanned, copied or duplicated, or posted to a publicly accessible website, in whole or in part.

4. Which theorist stated, "Grief results when an individual experiences a disruption in attachment to a love object"?

   a. Bowlby

   b. Worden

   c. Engle

   d. Lindemann

5. Which phrase best describes a person who has experienced a loss and subsequently does not experience the emotions associated with grief or does not demonstrate the typical behaviors associated with grief?

   a. Uncomplicated grief

   b. Dysfunctional grief

   c. Anticipatory grief

   d. Normal grief

6. An infant is brought by ambulance to the hospital and is not breathing. Which nursing outcome should the nurse plan to meet with the clients initially?

   a. Verbalizing feelings of grief

   b. Sharing grief with significant others

   c. Accepting the loss

   d. Renewing activities and relationships

7. Which statement by the client would indicate dysfunctional grieving?

   a. "I have no appetite."

   b. "This is my fault."

   c. "All I do is cry."

   d. "I have been depressed over my husband's death for a year."

8. Which nursing intervention is appropriate for a 4-year-old child who has recently experienced the death of a parent?

   a. Take the child to the cemetery.

   b. Reassure the child that the child did not contribute to the cause of death.

   c. Tell the child that the fear of death is irrational.

   d. Tell the child the parent is in "a kind of sleep."

© 2011 Cengage Learning. All Rights Reserved. May not be scanned, copied or duplicated, or posted to a publicly accessible website, in whole or in part.

9. A client is hospitalized with bowel cancer. The client's husband is angry and complaining of substandard care. How should the nurse respond to the husband?

    a. "I understand that you want the best for your wife. Tell me what it is that is bothering you about her care."

    b. "I know it is difficult for both you and your wife, but we are doing the best we can."

    c. "I apologize. We have been understaffed for the past 2 days."

    d. "I will contact the charge nurse and we will discuss this matter."

10. A 6-year-old child is dying of leukemia. The child's mother is having difficulty sleeping, cannot eat, and expresses guilt for "smoking while pregnant." The mother blames herself for her child's illness. Which nursing diagnosis is most appropriate for the mother?

    a. *Grieving*

    b. *Anticipatory grieving*

    c. *Dysfunctional grieving*

    d. *Distorted grief*

11. Match the Kübler-Ross stage of death and dying in the left column with an example of a client's statement or behavior from the right column that best exemplifies the stage.

    _____   denial   a. The client arranges his own wake and funeral.

    _____   anger   b. The client wants to be left alone.

    _____   bargaining   c. A client states, "Doctor, I want to live long enough to see my daughter get married."

    _____   depression   d. A client diagnosed with heart failure continues to eat foods high in sodium and cholesterol.

    _____   acceptance   e. A client states, "You don't know anything about taking care of someone like me."

12. A client who is dying demonstrates signs of depression. What is the purpose of depression in a dying client?

    a. It assists the client to regain control.

    b. It helps the client detach from life and become able to accept death.

    c. It helps the client postpone the inevitable.

    d. It is a tool for coping.

© 2011 Cengage Learning. All Rights Reserved. May not be scanned, copied or duplicated, or posted to a publicly accessible website, in whole or in part.

13. Which information would be most important to know in order to plan for the care of a dying client?

    a. The availability of a support system

    b. The client's oxygenation status

    c. The client's hydration status

    d. The availability of hospice care

14. Which need in Maslow's hierarchy of needs is a priority when caring for a dying client?

    a. Physiological needs

    b. Self-esteem needs

    c. Self-actualization needs

    d. Love and belonging needs

15. How should pain medication be administered to a client who is dying?

    a. Around the clock

    b. As needed

    c. When requested

    d. Prior to painful care or procedures

16. Match the physiological change after death in the left column with the nursing care implication in the right column.

    _____ algor mortis   a. The head should be elevated.

    _____ liver mortis   b. Carefully remove tape and dressing materials from the body.

    _____ rigor mortis   c. Dentures should be inserted, the eyes closed, and the body positioned soon after death.

17. Which is the greatest fear of dying clients?

    a. Loss of independence

    b. Loss of mobility

    c. Pain

    d. Dying alone

© 2011 Cengage Learning. All Rights Reserved. May not be scanned, copied or duplicated, or posted to a publicly accessible website, in whole or in part.

18. In which situation would an autopsy need to be performed after the death of a client?

   a. Elderly client with a history of chronic renal disease

   b. Client with a 5-year history of cancer treatment

   c. Middle-aged client who died at home unexpectedly

   d. Young male with a history of leukemia and hemophilia

19. Palliative care _____.

   a. focuses on attending to the reality of the client's loss.

   b. focuses on alleviating discomfort.

   c. focuses on supporting the family after their loss.

20. A client has been discharged to home to die. What should the family do to support social interaction with the client?

   a. Keep the room dimly lit.

   b. Play soft music around the clock.

   c. Provide meaningful stimuli for the client such as the newspaper or television.

   d. Leave the client alone and minimize intrusions.

Critical Thinking

21. Discuss Lindemann's theory of grief.

22. Explain how an unexpected or traumatic death can lead to dysfunctional grieving.

Activities

23. Divide the class into small groups, and discuss personal experiences with loss and death. Loss and death can mean many things to many people. It could mean the loss of a significant other, parent, sibling, aunt, uncle, or other extended family member. It could also mean the loss of a pet, friend, or object. Discuss the feelings that occurred after the realization of the loss or death. Attempt to identify the stages of grieving experienced.

24. Invite grief counselors or individuals who support crisis hotline centers to the classroom. Be prepared with questions to address how the counselors or crisis support individuals help others work through issues surrounding loss and death.

© 2011 Cengage Learning. All Rights Reserved. May not be scanned, copied or duplicated, or posted to a publicly accessible website, in whole or in part.

25. If possible, schedule a session to observe an autopsy. This could occur at a local teaching hospital or a county coroner's facility. Answer the following questions:

    a. What was the cause of death?

    b. What was the person's religious affiliation (if any)?

    c. What purpose will the autopsy serve?

    d. Did the person have any chronic illnesses?

    At the end of the autopsy experience, schedule a debriefing session to discuss feelings and impressions of the procedure, the behaviors of those conducting the autopsy, and the findings (if available). Ensure that all in attendance have an opportunity to discuss the experience.

© 2011 Cengage Learning. All Rights Reserved. May not be scanned, copied or duplicated, or posted to a publicly accessible website, in whole or in part.

Chapter 26 Vital Signs

1. Which data would be of the greatest concern to the nurse upon completion of the nursing admission assessment of a 70-year-old client with a diagnosis of pneumonia?

   a. Blood pressure 140/90

   b. Alert and oriented to date, time, and place

   c. Circumoral cyanosis and capillary refill greater than 3 seconds

   d. Frequently irregular pulse

2. Match the term in the left column with its definition from the right column.

   _____ hemodynamic regulation   a. The phase in which the ventricles contract to eject blood

   _____ systole   b. The measurement of pressure pulsations exerted against the blood vessel walls during systole and diastole

   _____ diastole   c. The maintenance of an appropriate environment in tissue fluids

   _____ stroke volume   d. The measurement of blood that enters the aorta with each ventricular contraction

   _____ cardiac output   e. The volume of blood pumped in 1 minute

   _____ pulse pressure   f. The phase in which ventricles are relaxed and no blood is being ejected

   _____ blood pressure   g. The measurement of the ratio of stroke volume to compliance of the arterial system

3. What is the normal pulse range for a 1-year-old infant?

   a. 60–80 bpm

   b. 80–110 bpm

   c. 80–170 bpm

   d. 100–200 bpm

© 2011 Cengage Learning. All Rights Reserved. May not be scanned, copied or duplicated, or posted to a publicly accessible website, in whole or in part.

4. A client tells the nurse that he takes digitalis once a day in the morning. Which vital sign change would the nurse expect to assess in this client?

   a. Increased blood pressure

   b. Decreased pulse rate

   c. Decreased respiratory rate

   d. Increased temperature

5. Which response is an effect of anxiety on the vital signs?

   a. Decreased temperature

   b. Decreased pulse

   c. Decreased respirations

   d. Increased blood pressure

6. Which route of temperature measurement is least accurate?

   a. Axillary

   b. Oral

   c. Tympanic

   d. Rectal

7. When discharging a client from the hospital after treatment for an acute hypertensive episode, the nurse recognizes the need for further teaching when the client makes which statement?

   a. "I'll walk every day."

   b. "I know I need to lose weight."

   c. "Drinking milk will help my high blood pressure."

   d. "Two medications for my blood pressure are too much medicine to take."

8. When environmental conditions produce an elevation in body temperature, diaphoresis results. This is an attempt to cool the body by which method of heat loss?

   a. Evaporation

   b. Convection

   c. Conduction

   d. Radiation

© 2011 Cengage Learning. All Rights Reserved. May not be scanned, copied or duplicated, or posted to a publicly accessible website, in whole or in part.

9. Which method is the proper technique to determine if a client is experiencing a pulse deficit?

   a. Simultaneously have one person count the apical pulse and another person count the radial pulse.

   b. Measure the apical pulse, wait 20–30 minutes, and remeasure the apical pulse rate.

   c. Measure the radial pulse in each arm and subtract the difference.

   d. Measure the distal pulse with a pulse oximeter and compare this to the apical heart rate.

10. The nurse is assessing a client's pulse by placing the stethoscope at the fifth intercostal space on the left side of the chest. The nurse is assessing is the _____ pulse.

   a. apical

   b. carotid

   c. brachial

   d. dorsalis pedis

11. Match the term in the left column with its definition from the right column.

   _____ eupnea   a. Shallow respirations

   _____ bradypnea   b. Easy respirations of a normal rate

   _____ hypoventilation   c. Deep rapid respirations

   _____ tachypnea   d. A respiratory rate of 10 or lower

   _____ hyperventilation   e. Thoracic breathing

   _____ diaphragmatic breathing   f. A respiratory rate of 24 or above

   _____ costal breathing   g. Breathing from the abdomen

   _____ dyspnea   h. Labored or forceful breathing, using accessory muscles in the chest and neck

12. The nurse needs to assess the blood pressure of a client who has an intravenous infusion in the left arm and an intermittent venous access device in the right hand. What should the nurse do?

   a. Use the left arm to assess blood pressure.

   b. Use the right arm to assess blood pressure.

   c. Document that the blood pressure cannot be obtained.

   d. Ask the prescribing practitioner to assess the client's blood pressure.

© 2011 Cengage Learning. All Rights Reserved. May not be scanned, copied or duplicated, or posted to a publicly accessible website, in whole or in part.

13. How long should a nurse wait to reassess a client's blood pressure in the same arm?

    a. 30 seconds

    b. 1 minute

    c. 2 minutes

    d. 3 minutes

14. What is the minimum length of time to wait before measuring the oral temperature of a client who has taken a drink of ice water?

    a. No wait is necessary.

    b. 5 minutes

    c. 15 minutes

    d. 45 minutes

15. High blood pressure in women can be attributed to

    a. birth control pills.

    b. exercise.

    c. normal weight.

    d. sex.

16. Which hemodynamic regulator for blood pressure control describes the thickness of the blood?

    a. Blood volume

    b. Cardiac output

    c. Peripheral vascular resistance

    d. Viscosity

17. The nurse assesses a client's weight to be 176 lb. This weight is equal to _____ kg.

18. A client is to have a daily weight. What should be done when implementing this order?

    a. Weigh the client when able.

    b. Weigh the client after morning care.

    c. Weigh the client on the same scale, with the same type of clothing, at the same time of day.

    d. Weigh the client before sleep.

© 2011 Cengage Learning. All Rights Reserved. May not be scanned, copied or duplicated, or posted to a publicly accessible website, in whole or in part.

19.   A client has a temperature reading that remains above normal with minimal variations of less than 1°. This client is exhibiting a(n) _____ fever.

    a.   intermittent

    b.   remittent

    c.   sustained

    d.   recurrent

20.   A 35-year-old client's heart rate is 110 beats per minute. This finding is considered

    a.   tachycardia.

    b.   bradycardia.

    c.   irregular.

    d.   arrhythmia.

Critical Thinking

21.   A client ambulates to the examination room, and the nurse assesses the blood pressure to be 150/90. Explain what the nurse should do.

22.   Explain how a client with a brain injury can develop an elevated temperature.

Activities

22.   Provide a sufficient number of thermometer devices, blood pressure cuffs, sphygmomanometers, and stethoscopes. Divide the group into pairs of two, and have each pair practice assessing vital signs on each other. When measuring temperature, measure the difference in temperature between oral and axillary and oral and tympanic. When measuring blood pressure, measure the pressure sitting and standing to detect differences with postural changes.

23.   Evaluate the accuracy of a variety of weight-measuring devices in the home, school, hospital, and community. Many department stores and pharmacies have scales to measure weight. Weigh yourself on a reliable scale, and document the weight. Then weigh yourself on a variety of different devices to assess the accuracy and fluctuation that exists. Attempt to follow the process as if prescribed daily weights while in the hospital—at the same time of day, wearing the same type of clothing. Discuss the variations in the weight-monitoring devices assessed. Discuss also how the variations in the weight-monitoring devices might alter a client's perception of his or her weight.

© 2011 Cengage Learning. All Rights Reserved. May not be scanned, copied or duplicated, or posted to a publicly accessible website, in whole or in part.

Chapter 27   Physical Assessment

1. In which position should the client be placed when the nurse is going to assess the abdomen and extremities?

   a. Sims'

   b. Prone

   c. Sitting

   d. Supine

2. In which order should the nurse assess a client's abdomen?

   _____   a.   Auscultation

   _____   b.   Percussion

   _____   c.   Palpation

   _____   d.   Inspection

3. The nurse assesses an indentation on a client's ankle region as being 6 mm. What does this finding reflect?

   a. +1 pitting edema

   b. +2 pitting edema

   c. +3 pitting edema

   d. +4 pitting edema

4. To which organ system does the documentation PERRLA refer?

   a. Eyes

   b. Ears

   c. Mouth

   d. Lungs

© 2011 Cengage Learning. All Rights Reserved. May not be scanned, copied or duplicated, or posted to a publicly accessible website, in whole or in part.

5. Match the term associated with respiratory assessment in the left column with its definition from the right column.

_____ stridor   a. Heard over predominantly the base of the lungs as a fine, high-pitched popping sound of short duration

_____ pleural friction rub   b. High-pitched musical sounds that can be heard over all the lung fields

_____ wheezes   c. A crowing sound heard predominantly on inspiration

_____ rhonchi   d. Accumulation of fluid in the interstitial and air spaces of the lung

_____ crackles   e. Accumulation of pus in the pleural cavity

6. Which finding is described as a fingernail to nail base angle of greater than 180°?

a. Normal nail

b. Clubbing

c. Spoon nail

d. Beau's line

7. Which of the following can be the cause of a grade II heart murmur?

a. Mitral regurgitation

b. A bundle branch block

c. Pneumothorax

d. Angina

8. What is the appropriate length of time a nurse should listen to accurately assess bowel sounds?

a. 15 seconds in each quadrant

b. 30 seconds in each quadrant

c. 45 seconds in each quadrant

d. 1 minute in each quadrant

9. It is documented that a client has petechiae on the arms and legs. Which statement describes how this finding appears upon assessment?

a. Purplish blue lesions with fading areas of green and yellow

b. Flat, round 1–3-mm lesions that are reddish-purple

c. Spiderlike lesions of varying size and bluish in color

d. Ruby red, round 1–3-mm lesions

© 2011 Cengage Learning. All Rights Reserved. May not be scanned, copied or duplicated, or posted to a publicly accessible website, in whole or in part.

10. Which assessment provides information about cerebellar function?

    a. Level of consciousness assessment data

    b. Assessment data regarding cranial nerve function

    c. Assessment of muscle tone and strength

    d. Assessment of the client's gait

11. The nurse places her hands on areas of the client's chest and asks the client to say "ninety-nine." What is the nurse doing?

    a. Palpating for tactile fremitus

    b. Palpating for lifts

    c. Palpating for heaves

    d. Palpating for edema

12. A bulging of the anterior vaginal wall due to the protrusion of the urinary bladder indicates a

_____.

13. Which heart valve is assessed by auscultating to the right of the sternum?

    a. Mitral

    b. Tricuspid

    c. Pulmonic

    d. Aortic

14. List the seven Fs of abdominal distention.

    F _____

    F _____

    F _____

    F _____

    F _____

    F _____

    F _____

© 2011 Cengage Learning. All Rights Reserved. May not be scanned, copied or duplicated, or posted to a publicly accessible website, in whole or in part.

15. The primary sound elicited when percussing the abdomen is

    a. dullness.

    b. bronchovesicular.

    c. vesicular.

    d. tympany.

16. Match the musculoskeletal status term with the correct definition.

    _____ a. hypertrophy   a. Thin, flabby muscles due to reduced muscle size and shape

    _____ b. atrophy   b. Increased muscle tone

    _____ c. hypertonicity   c. Flabby muscle with poor tone

    _____ d. hypotonicity   d. Increase in muscle size and shape due to an increase in muscle fiber

17. The nurse who asks a client to close his eyes, places a key in his hand, and asks the client to identify the object is assessing for _____.

18. The nurse has a client sit on the edge of the bed with the legs dangling and taps the knee area to elicit a response. Which deep tendon reflex is the nurse assessing?

    a. Biceps

    b. Brachioradialis

    c. Patellar

    d. Plantar

19. The nurse is documenting that a client's reflexes are normal. Which symbol would indicate this finding?

    a. 0

    b. +

    c. ++

    d. +++

20. Which population experiences the highest incidence of prostate cancer?

    a. African Americans

    b. Caucasians

    c. Hispanics

    d. American Indians

© 2011 Cengage Learning. All Rights Reserved. May not be scanned, copied or duplicated, or posted to a publicly accessible website, in whole or in part.

Critical Thinking

21. What should be assessed during the general survey of a client?

22. Discuss the senses that the nurse uses when assessing a client.

Activities

23. Practice the technique of percussion by eliciting sounds from a variety of objects such as a desk, the wall, a plastic cup, and a variety of body parts such as the thigh area, abdominal region, and lungs.

24. Plan to practice the assessment of each of the major body systems. This practice could occur in a laboratory setting or the clinical environment. If in the clinical setting, divide the class into groups of two students and provide each group with a guide sheet to assist with the flow of the physical assessment. Conduct the physical assessment and document findings. At the conclusion of each pair of assessments, discuss the findings and what the findings could suggest.

25. Practice using a variety of assessment tools to increase confidence and proficiency such as a reflex hammer, a Snellen chart, cotton swabs, safety pins, and a tape measure.

© 2011 Cengage Learning. All Rights Reserved. May not be scanned, copied or duplicated, or posted to a publicly accessible website, in whole or in part.

Chapter 28   Diagnostic Testing

1. Which term expresses a laboratory test's ability to correctly identify individuals who have a disease?

    a. Specificity

    b. Sensitivity

    c. Incidence

    d. Predictive value

2. Which of the following can cause hemoconcentration?

    a. Prolonged application of a tourniquet during venipuncture

    b. Bedrest

    c. Diabetes

    d. Gallbladder disease

3. Which method is considered most reliable when identifying a client prior to a diagnostic procedure?

    a. Asking the client to state his or her name

    b. Checking the arm or leg band

    c. Asking a family member the client's name

    d. Checking the chart that accompanies the client

4. What should be done prior to performing an arterial puncture on a client?

    a. Measure the blood pressure.

    b. Assess the pulse.

    c. Conduct the Allen's test.

    d. Apply a tourniquet.

© 2011 Cengage Learning. All Rights Reserved. May not be scanned, copied or duplicated, or posted to a publicly accessible website, in whole or in part.

5. What puncture type is preferred to assess a client's blood glucose level?

   a. Venipuncture

   b. Arterial puncture

   c. Capillary puncture

   d. None of the above

6. The nurse needs to collect a urine sample for culture. Which collection method provides a sterile specimen?

   a. Random collection

   b. Timed collection

   c. Clean-voided specimen

   d. Collection from a closed urinary drainage system

7. A client is receiving a respiratory nebulizer treatment every 4 hours and has an order that reads "arterial blood gases post nebulizer treatment." When should the blood gases be drawn?

   a. Immediately after the treatment

   b. 15 minutes after the treatment

   c. 20 minutes after the treatment

   d. Immediately before the next treatment

8. What is the purpose of routine heparin solution instillation in an unused port of a central line catheter?

   a. To prevent blood clots from forming in the catheter lumen

   b. To prevent the growth of microorganisms in the tubing

   c. To prevent analytes from forming in the tubing

   d. To prevent clotting in the specimen obtained from the port

9. What should be done with the first void of a 24-hour urine specimen?

   a. Discard it.

   b. Place it in the collection canister.

   c. Send it for culture.

   d. Send it for routine analysis.

© 2011 Cengage Learning. All Rights Reserved. May not be scanned, copied or duplicated, or posted to a publicly accessible website, in whole or in part.

10. Which drug decreases the prothrombin time (PT)?

   a. Salicylates

   b. Steroids

   c. Digitalis

   d. Dilantin

11. Which of the following diagnostic tests measures the intrinsic clotting mechanism factors (I, II, V, XI, XII)?

   a. PTT

   b. PT

   c. Thrombin time

12. Which is a plasma protein that requires vitamin K for synthesis?

   a. Prothrombin

   b. Thrombin

   c. Fibrinogen

   d. Platelets

13. The prescribing practitioner orders a "CBC with differential." When you are filling out the lab slip, which of the following should you check off?

   a. CBC and lymphocytes

   b. CBC and platelets

   c. CBC and monocytes

   d. CBC and WBC

14. Which of the following would a low hemoglobin and low hematocrit level indicate?

   a. Anemia

   b. Hemorrhage

   c. Hodgkin's disease

   d. Hypothyroidism

© 2011 Cengage Learning. All Rights Reserved. May not be scanned, copied or duplicated, or posted to a publicly accessible website, in whole or in part.

15. When a client is to receive blood, a type and crossmatch are performed. What is the purpose of the crossmatch procedure?

    a. To determine the presence or absence of A or B antigens in the client's blood

    b. To determine if the Rh factor is present in the client's blood

    c. To determine the compatibility of the recipient's blood with the donor blood

    d. To determine if the Rh agglutinins are present in the donor blood

16. A client is having a hemoglobin electrophoresis conducted. Which disease process does the nurse realize this laboratory test is used to diagnose?

    a. Renal failure

    b. Leukemia

    c. Arthritis

    d. Sickle cell disease

17. The laboratory values for a client show an elevated LDH_1 and an elevated CPK_2 (MB). This is indicative of

    a. myocardial damage.

    b. liver damage.

    c. brain damage.

    d. kidney damage.

18. Which laboratory value is normal for an adult client?

    a. Sodium 142 mEq/L

    b. Potassium 6.5 mEq/L

    c. Chloride 100 mEq/L

    d. Magnesium 1.6 mEq/L

19. A client's ESR (erythrocyte sedimentation rate) is moderately elevated. What does this elevation most likely indicate?

    a. A concomitant elevation in blood glucose

    b. Increased stomach acidity

    c. The presence of an inflammatory process

    d. A folic acid deficiency

© 2011 Cengage Learning. All Rights Reserved. May not be scanned, copied or duplicated, or posted to a publicly accessible website, in whole or in part.

20. Match the study in the left column with the organ or body system it examines in the right column.

_____	angiography	a.	Peritoneal cavity
_____	lymphangiography	b.	Heart
_____	cholangiography	c.	Blood vessels
_____	cystography	d.	Lymphatic system
_____	intravenous pyelogram	e.	Urinary system
_____	myelography	f.	Bladder
_____	electrocardiogram	g.	Biliary system
_____	arthroscopy	h.	Spinal cord
_____	laparoscopy	i.	Joint structures
_____	proctosigmoidoscopy	j.	Rectum and colon

21. A sexually active female college student seeks counseling for the prevention of sexually transmitted diseases. Which screening measure should the nurse recommend? (Select all that apply.)

   a. Mammogram

   b. Pap test

   c. Cervical cytology for HPV

   d. Prophylactic antibiotics

Critical Thinking

22. Explain the difference between LDL cholesterol and HDL cholesterol.

23. Discuss what type of teaching should be provided for a client before a diagnostic test.

© 2011 Cengage Learning. All Rights Reserved. May not be scanned, copied or duplicated, or posted to a publicly accessible website, in whole or in part.

Activities

24. Accompany a phlebotomist to collect blood specimens. Observe the technique used by the phlebotomist to include identification of client, application of gloves, care of sharps, selection of collection tubes, technique used to collect blood, client care, disposal of sharps, and hand hygiene after each collection.

25. Provide a variety of blood glucose monitoring devices. Have antiseptic swabs, cotton, gauze pads, testing strips, gloves, and sterile lancets. Divide the class into groups of two, and have the groups practice conducting a blood glucose test on each other. Discuss the experience in a large group when the testing is done.

26. Provide a selection of specimen collection devices for analysis. Have available collection devices for urine, stool, and sputum. Discuss the challenges when using these collection devices. In particular, what will need to be done if the device must be kept sterile?

© 2011 Cengage Learning. All Rights Reserved. May not be scanned, copied or duplicated, or posted to a publicly accessible website, in whole or in part.

Chapter 29 Safety, Infection Control, and Hygiene

1. Match the terms in the left column with their definitions from the right column.

   _____ pathogenicity

   _____ pathogens

   _____ virulence

   _____ infection

   _____ resident floras

   _____ transient floras

   _____ host

   _____ agent

   a. Bacteria, viruses, fungi, protozoa, *Rickettsia*

   b. Something that is capable of causing disease

   c. A plant or animal that harbors and provides sustenance for another organism

   d. Microorganisms acquired from environmental contact

   e. The degree to which a pathogen can produce disease

   f. Ability of a microorganism to produce disease

   g. Invasion of a body tissue by microorganisms that results in cellular injury

   h. Always present, usually nonharmful microorganisms

2. Match each term in the left column with its definition from the right column.

   _____ antigen

   _____ antibody

   _____ lymphokine

   _____ humoral immunity

   _____ acquired immunity

   a. Released by T cells; attracts phagocytes and lymphocytes

   b. Protein substance that counteracts the effects of autogenic toxins

   c. A substance that causes an antibody to form

   d. Stimulation of B cells and antibody production

   e. The formation of memory B cells; protects the host from the invasion of microbes

3. The Joint Commission National Patient Safety Goals include all of the following *except*

   a. ask clients to identify themselves routinely.

   b. improve staff communication.

   c. prevent infection.

   d. prevent clients from falling.

© 2011 Cengage Learning. All Rights Reserved. May not be scanned, copied or duplicated, or posted to a publicly accessible website, in whole or in part.

4. Which of the following infections are health care workers most at risk to acquire?

    a. HIV

    b. HCV

    c. Lyme disease

    d. Abscess

5. The percentage of adults in the United States over 65 who suffer falls is

    a. 25%.

    b. 33%.

    c. 10%.

    d. 20%.

6. What do the microorganisms VRE and MRSA have in common?

    a. They are transmitted only in the droplet form.

    b. They are common drug-resistant nosocomial infections.

    c. They are uropathogens.

    d. They tend to invade immune-intact hosts.

7. The nurse develops a rash around the wrists and on the back of the hands that might be allergic contact dermatitis from latex gloves. What should the nurse do?

    a. Avoid direct contact with latex-containing products until further evaluated by a prescribing practitioner.

    b. Continue to use latex-containing products and follow up with good handwashing.

    c. Ingest antiallergic medication before using latex-containing products.

    d. Wear nonlatex gloves at all times when delivering client care.

8. Which of the following describes the first stage of the inflammatory process?

    a. Increased blood flow to the damaged area

    b. Infiltration of leukocytes into the damaged area

    c. Leakage of large amounts of plasma into the damaged area

    d. Release of chemicals

9. Two methods of practicing hand hygiene are _____ and _____.

© 2011 Cengage Learning. All Rights Reserved. May not be scanned, copied or duplicated, or posted to a publicly accessible website, in whole or in part.

10. The main method of preventing the transmission of MRSA is

    a. medical asepsis.

    b. standard precautions.

    c. handwashing.

    d. powder-free gloves.

11. A client is suspected of having an infection. Which test result would indicate that an infection is present in the client?

    a. Elevated neutrophils

    b. Normal lymphocytes

    c. Increased monocytes

    d. Low white blood cell count

12. Which of the following nursing interventions is a priority for a client at risk for falls?

    a. Provide adequate hydration and nutrition.

    b. Keep the bed in the lowest possible position.

    c. Place the patient in a room near the nurses' station.

    d. Offer the bedpan every 2 hours while the patient is in bed.

13. A client with respiratory symptoms is placed on droplet precautions. Which procedures are included in these precautions?

    a. Gloves and gowns when in contact with the client

    b. Gloves, gowns, and the use of a mask within 3 feet of the client

    c. A private room and use of a HEPA filter mask when in the client's room

    d. A private room and the use of a mask within 3 feet of the client

14. Place the following steps of bathing an adult in sequence from the beginning to the end of the bath.

    _____ Document skin assessment, type of bath, and client response.

    _____ Wash back.

    _____ Apply lotion or powder, then gown.

    _____ Place bath blanket over client.

    _____ Wash face.

    _____ Wash arms and hands.

    _____ Wash perineal area.

    _____ Wash legs and feet.

    _____ Wash chest and abdomen.

    _____ Obtain bath water.

© 2011 Cengage Learning. All Rights Reserved. May not be scanned, copied or duplicated, or posted to a publicly accessible website, in whole or in part.

15. Which action would the nurse take to prevent the spread of infection by a client with a productive cough?

    a. Provide a HEPA filter mask.

    b. Place the client on droplet precautions.

    c. Provide tissues and have client use them when coughing.

    d. Monitor the client's temperature every 4 hours.

16. List the three reasons to use restraints.

    a. _____

    b. _____

    c. _____

17. Which drug is a commonly used chemical restraint?

    a. Acetaminophen

    b. Salicylic acid

    c. Digoxin

    d. Anxiolytics

18. The type of fire extinguisher that can be used for any type of fire is

    a. A.

    b. B and C.

    c. A, B, and C.

    d. D.

19. Match the term to the correct definition.

    _____ a. cleansing   a. Total elimination of all microorganisms

    _____ b. disinfection   b. Removal of soil or organic material

    _____ c. sterilization   c. Elimination of pathogens except spores

20. A male client on anticoagulant therapy asks to be shaved. What should the nurse do?

    a. Shave the client with a straight razor.

    b. Shave the client with a safety razor.

    c. Shave the client with an electric razor.

    d. Counsel the client to grow a beard and mustache.

© 2011 Cengage Learning. All Rights Reserved. May not be scanned, copied or duplicated, or posted to a publicly accessible website, in whole or in part.

Critical Thinking

21. Explain what a nurse can do to reduce the feelings of isolation and loneliness in a client requiring isolation precautions.

22. Discuss the implications of the Medicare Modernization Act.

Activities

23. Access the Centers for Disease Control and Prevention Web site at http://www.cdc.gov. Click on the link Workplace Safety & Health. Under Top Workplace Health Links, scroll down to and click on Healthcare Workers. Review the topics on this page. Read the information under Related Sites, CDC Topics, Infection Control in Healthcare Settings. This is another Web page with many additional links, specifically Infection Control Topics and Infection Control Resources. Discuss the importance of infection control in the health care setting and ways to ensure infection control principles are maintained when providing client care.

24. In the laboratory or clinical area, practice making an unoccupied bed and an occupied bed. If in the laboratory, have another student serve as the client when practicing the occupied bed process.

25. Invite hospital infection control nurses and nurses from the community Department of Public Health to the class to discuss the most prevalent infectious diseases being seen or reported today. Prepare to discuss ways in which the transmission of these diseases can be reduced and what efforts are currently under way to reduce or eliminate these diseases from society.

© 2011 Cengage Learning. All Rights Reserved. May not be scanned, copied or duplicated, or posted to a publicly accessible website, in whole or in part.

Chapter 30 Medication Administration

1. A "prescribing practitioner" refers to
   a. advanced practice nurses.
   b. dentists.
   c. physicians.
   d. all of the above.

2. Which mandate established the United States Pharmacopeia (USP) and the National Formulary (NF) as the official bodies that establish drug standards in the United States?
   a. The Harrison Narcotic Act
   b. The Food, Drug, and Cosmetic Act
   c. The Pure Food and Drug Act
   d. The Kefauver-Harris Act

3. Which medication is considered a schedule C-1 controlled substance?
   a. Heroin
   b. Amphetamines
   c. Nonamphetamine stimulants
   d. Sedatives

4. _____ refers to the movement of drugs from the blood into various body fluids and tissues.

5. Match each term in the left column with its definition from the right column.

   _____ peak plasma level   a. Maintenance blood level of a drug

   _____ onset of action   b. When the body begins to respond to a drug

   _____ drug plateau   c. Highest blood concentration level of a drug

   _____ drug half-life   d. The time it takes the body to eliminate half of the blood concentration of a drug

© 2011 Cengage Learning. All Rights Reserved. May not be scanned, copied or duplicated, or posted to a publicly accessible website, in whole or in part.

6. What instructions should be provided to a client being given a sublingual medication?

   a. Chew the medication before swallowing.

   b. Wait a few minutes before eating or drinking anything.

   c. Swallow the medication whole.

   d. Dissolve this medication completely and swallow quickly.

7. The medication order reads: heparin 5000 units subcutaneous b.i.d. Where in the body will this medication be given?

   a. The dermis

   b. The muscle

   c. The fatty tissue

   d. The vein

8. Identify the medication order incorrectly written.

   a. Pepcid 20 mg PO q.d.

   b. Colace 100 mg PO b.i.d.

   c. Demerol 50.0 mg IM q4 hours prn

   d. Thyroxin 25 mcg PO q am

9. Which term is defined as something that occurs when the body cannot metabolize a drug, causing the drug to accumulate in the blood?

   a. Drug tolerance

   b. Toxic effect

   c. Idiosyncratic reaction

   d. Adverse reaction

10. A client is prescribed Coumadin. How should the nurse instruct this client?

    a. This medication can lead to vitamin D deficiency.

    b. This medication can cause vitamin C deficiency.

    c. Do not take this medication with high-acid fruit or vegetable juices.

    d. Limit foods high in vitamin K, such as green leafy vegetables.

© 2011 Cengage Learning. All Rights Reserved. May not be scanned, copied or duplicated, or posted to a publicly accessible website, in whole or in part.

11. Mrs. Kaplan is ordered dorzolamide hydrochloride 1 gtt each eye t.i.d. Where and when will you administer this medication?

 a.   In the right eye, twice per day

 b.   In both eyes, twice per day

 c.   In the left eye, three times per day

 d.   In both eyes, three times per day

12. The nurse needs to administer Tylenol 1 tsp q4h prn for a temperature above 101°F. The medication cup is marked in milliliters. How many milliliters should the nurse pour?

 a.   2 mL

 b.   5 mL

 c.   10 mL

 d.   15 mL

13. Medications that may be given via a gastric or nasogastric tube are

 a.   subcutaneous.

 b.   oral.

 c.   enteric coated.

 d.   sustained released.

14. A medication order is as follows: Inapsine 0.625 mg IV push q 4–6h prn nausea/vomiting. The medication comes supplied as 2.5 mg/mL. How much should the nurse give to a client needing a dose?

 a.   0.25 mL

 b.   0.50 mL

 c.   1.0 mL

 d.   1.5 mL

15. List the five rights of medication administration.

 a.   _____

 b.   _____

 c.   _____

 d.   _____

 e.   _____

© 2011 Cengage Learning. All Rights Reserved. May not be scanned, copied or duplicated, or posted to a publicly accessible website, in whole or in part.

16. The nurse finds medications at a client's bedside. What should the nurse do?

    a. Provide the medications to the client.

    b. Remove the medications and discard.

    c. Confirm all of the medications with the MAR before administering.

    d. Report a medication error and contact the prescribing practitioner.

17. A client is to receive all medications through a PEG tube. The MAR reads: Enteric-coated ASA 1 tablet q.d. via tube. What should the nurse do?

    a. Crush the tablet, dissolve it, and administer via the PEG tube.

    b. Call the pharmacy to see if a liquid substitution is available.

    c. Contact the prescribing practitioner to clarify the order.

    d. Substitute with uncoated aspirin and provide the medication through the tube.

18. Which needle gauge represents the largest needle diameter?

    a. 25 gauge

    b. 20 gauge

    c. 19 gauge

19. The MAR reads: Neupogen 300 mcg subcutaneous q.d. Neupogen is supplied as 300 mcg/mL. Which syringe should be used to administer this medication?

    a. 1-mL tuberculin syringe with a 27-gauge needle

    b. 3-mL hypodermic syringe with a 20-gauge needle

    c. 3-mL hypodermic syringe with a 25-gauge needle

    d. 0.5-mL hypodermic syringe with a 27-gauge needle

20. When administering an intramuscular injection to a client, blood appears in the syringe. What should the nurse do?

    a. Remove the needle and discard the medication.

    b. Continue to give the medication.

    c. Withdraw the needle and reinsert after applying a new needle to the syringe.

    d. Administer as rapidly as possible.

© 2011 Cengage Learning. All Rights Reserved. May not be scanned, copied or duplicated, or posted to a publicly accessible website, in whole or in part.

21. What is the largest volume that can be injected into a large muscle of an adult?

  a. 1 cc

  b. 2 cc

  c. 3 cc

  d. 4 cc

22. From which container would a filtered needle be indicated to withdraw medication?

  a. Ampule

  b. Multidose vial

  c. Single-dose vial

  d. Prefilled syringe

23. When administering an IV piggyback medication through a gravity flow system, the primary solution bag is lowered, via extension hook, prior to the start of the medication infusion. What is the rationale for this action?

  a. Ensures that no air will enter the secondary set tubing

  b. Reduces the risk of microorganisms entering the primary line tubing

  c. Allows the primary solution to continue infusing during the medication administration

  d. An increased hydrostatic pressure in the secondary bag causes the primary solution to stop flowing

24. Which nursing consideration is critical when delivering medications via IV push?

  a. The time interval to inject the drug

  b. The port of the IV tubing used to place the medication

  c. The time it takes for the drug to be absorbed

  d. The age of the client

25. A client asks why a metered-dose inhaler needs to be shaken before use. How should the nurse respond to this client?

  a. "It makes sure that the two medications are mixed properly."

  b. "It activates the medication."

  c. "It allows for the medication to mix with the aerosol propellant."

  d. "It gets into the lungs faster."

© 2011 Cengage Learning. All Rights Reserved. May not be scanned, copied or duplicated, or posted to a publicly accessible website, in whole or in part.

Critical Thinking

26. If a nurse is working in a health care organization that has a sixth medication right, such as the right documentation, what does this mean?

27. Describe characteristics of a drug-impaired nurse in the workplace.

Activities

28. Practice holding and using a variety of syringe sizes, such as tuberculin, insulin, and subcutaneous/intramuscular. Practice filling the syringes with sterile water from vials. Consider the need to maintain standard precautions when preparing medications for injection.

29. Invite a panel of pharmacists to the classroom to discuss dispensing medications to clients. The pharmacists can be from surrounding health care facilities as well as community pharmacies. What challenges do pharmacists face when working with health care professionals? What challenges do pharmacists face when working directly with clients?

30. The administration of medications is a skill that improves with practice and proficiency. Practice preparing medications by following the five rights of medication administration. Research the medication's purpose, recommended dose, routes, and expected actions prior to administration.

© 2011 Cengage Learning. All Rights Reserved. May not be scanned, copied or duplicated, or posted to a publicly accessible website, in whole or in part.

Chapter 31 Complementary and Alternative Modalities

1. Ayurvedic medicine embraces the concept of *prana*. Prana is best thought of as a

   a. meditative practice.

   b. life force or energy.

   c. transport system for body energy.

   d. healing remedy.

2. The field of science that studies the relationship between the cognitive, affective, and physical aspects of humans is called

   a. neuroanatomy.

   b. psychoneuroimmunology.

   c. neurophysiology.

   d. psychobiology.

3. Which group of physiological responses reflects the benefits of meditation?

   a. Increased oxygen consumption, increased heart rate, and increased blood pressure

   b. Decreased oxygen consumption, decreased heart rate, and decreased blood pressure

   c. Alteration in immune system function, increased levels of lactic acid, and decreased blood pressure

   d. Alteration in immune system function, increased levels of lactic acid, and increased blood pressure

4. Which perspective on the practice of medicine would emphasize health maintenance and disease prevention through lifestyle choice?

   a. Alternative medicine

   b. Allopathic medicine

   c. Traditional medicine

   d. Western medicine

© 2011 Cengage Learning. All Rights Reserved. May not be scanned, copied or duplicated, or posted to a publicly accessible website, in whole or in part.

5. Which statement best describes the goal of the nurse when the nurse serves as an instrument of healing? The goal is to

    a. provide therapeutic touch to clients when needed.

    b. dispense medicinal herbs useful for a wide variety of ailments.

    c. help the client draw upon inner resources for healing to occur.

    d. help the client access the life force energy in order to facilitate healing.

6. _____ is a type of thinking without words in which the senses are used to evoke one's imagination.

7. Which of the following complementary/alternative interventions is considered a body-movement intervention?

    a. Tai chi

    b. Imagery

    c. Acupuncture

    d. Aromatherapy

8. Which best describes the physiological source of the relaxation response?

    a. Increased arousal of the sympathetic system

    b. Increased arousal of the parasympathetic system

    c. Suppression of the parasympathetic system

    d. Suppression of the sympathetic system

9. Sequence the following therapeutic touch (TT) phases in order from the beginning of an intervention to the end of an intervention.

    _____ Evaluation

    _____ Unruffling

    _____ Scanning

    _____ Centering

    _____ Balancing, rebalancing

© 2011 Cengage Learning. All Rights Reserved. May not be scanned, copied or duplicated, or posted to a publicly accessible website, in whole or in part.

10. In both therapeutic touch and healing touch, the practitioner uses centering before initiating treatment. Which best describes the process of centering? Centering is

   a. a process of bringing body, mind, and emotions to a quiet, focused state of consciousness.

   b. a process of focusing attention on a client.

   c. a process whereby the emotional involvement between the practitioner and client is genuine and purposeful.

   d. a process whereby the practitioner directs energy toward the client.

11. The massage technique in which the whole hand is used to provide firm, gliding, even-pressured strokes is called

   a. effleurage.

   b. petrissage.

   c. tapotement.

   d. vibration.

12. The goal of mindful meditation is to

   a. relieve stress.

   b. depress the immune system.

   c. regulate vital signs.

   d. control mood.

13. The underlying principle of chiropractic therapy is to

   a. reduce muscle tension.

   b. improve blood flow.

   c. remove blocks to nerve signals sent by the brain to the body.

   d. restore the client to harmony with nature and the universe.

14. The last step in the process of healing touch is

   a. grounding.

   b. documentation.

   c. intervention.

   d. centering.

© 2011 Cengage Learning. All Rights Reserved. May not be scanned, copied or duplicated, or posted to a publicly accessible website, in whole or in part.

15. Which food is a source of phytoestrogens?

    a. Green tea

    b. Tomatoes

    c. Onions

    d. Soybeans

16. An unstable molecule that alters genetic codes and triggers the development of cancer cells is a(n)

    a. antioxidant.

    b. free radical.

    c. phytochemical.

    d. neuropeptide.

17. Identify the herb that is believed to have medicinal value for the treatment of mild to moderate depression.

    a. Ginger

    b. Thyme

    c. Feverfew

    d. St. John's wort

18. Which herbal product, when combined with Coumadin, increases the risk of bleeding?

    a. Licorice root

    b. Danshen

    c. Belladonna

    d. Ginkgo biloba

19. The practice of tai chi has helped individuals experiencing

    a. heart disease.

    b. depression.

    c. fibromyalgia.

    d. cancer.

20. The therapeutic use of concentrated oils extracted from plants and flowers is considered _____.

© 2011 Cengage Learning. All Rights Reserved. May not be scanned, copied or duplicated, or posted to a publicly accessible website, in whole or in part.

Critical Thinking

21.   Explain why a client who sees an acupuncturist for headache relief does not want his prescribing practitioner to know about the treatments.

22.   A client tells the nurse that she wears inserts in her shoes that provide relaxing massage to her feet throughout the day. Explain how these inserts might be similar to the alternative medicine approach of reflexology.

Activities

23.   Access the National Center for Complementary and Alternative Medicine Web site at http://nccam.nih.gov. Review the information under the link Take Charge of Your Health. Then, access the Training Link and click on Online Lectures, where you will find a variety of continuing education programs for review. Review one program and prepare to discuss the information learned with others in the class.

24.   Locate a vitamin and herbal supplement store in the community. Go to the store and see the different types of vitamins and herbal supplements available. Make a list of vitamins and herbal supplements, and research their uses. Discuss the information learned with others in the class.

25.   Contact a local community college or trade school that instructs students in massage therapy. Invite an instructor or several students from this facility to come to the classroom and review the process of massage with the class.

© 2011 Cengage Learning. All Rights Reserved. May not be scanned, copied or duplicated, or posted to a publicly accessible website, in whole or in part.

Chapter 32   Oxygenation

1. A client has an oxygen saturation of 90% on 4 L of oxygen via nasal cannula. The nurse would interpret this finding as

   a. within normal limits.

   b. too high.

   c. too low for a client receiving oxygen.

   d. an indicator of pending respiratory arrest; preventive measures need to be implemented immediately.

2. The highest possible concentration of oxygen will require the use of which delivery system?

   a. Face mask

   b. Venturi mask

   c. Nasal cannula

   d. Mask with a reservoir bag

3. A client who experiences a collection of blood in the pleural space is experiencing which of the following conditions?

   a. Pneumothorax

   b. Pleural effusion

   c. Chylothorax

   d. Hemothorax

4. Pulse oximetry measures _____ via light waves.

5. Which medication would be indicated to promote bronchial dilation and increase ciliary movement?

   a. Cromolyn sodium

   b. Aminophylline

   c. Beclomethasone

   d. Mucomyst

© 2011 Cengage Learning. All Rights Reserved. May not be scanned, copied or duplicated, or posted to a publicly accessible website, in whole or in part.

6. A client with a history of chronic obstructive pulmonary disease and chest pain is admitted to the intensive care unit to rule out a myocardial infarction. Which test would determine the extent to which the client is experiencing air trapping?

    a. Sputum sample analysis

    b. Arterial blood gas analysis

    c. Electrocardiography

    d. Ventilation scan

7. Clubbing is a physical assessment finding that indicates

    a. ventilation/perfusion mismatch.

    b. atelectasis.

    c. chronic hypoxia.

    d. chronic hypoxemia.

8. Through which structure does freshly oxygenated blood return to the heart in preparation for entering the general circulation?

    a. Pulmonary artery

    b. Pulmonary vein

    c. Capillaries

    d. Left ventricle

9. A client comes to the emergency department complaining of right lower chest pain and shortness of breath. Which question should be asked during the focal interview to provide the most information about the client's problem?

    a. "How many packs of cigarettes a day do you smoke?"

    b. "Describe the pain for me."

    c. "Tell me what you have had to eat today."

    d. "Can you describe your medical history?"

10. Which assessment finding indicates that a client needs to be suctioned?

    a. Diminished breath sounds

    b. Inability to perform deep breathing and coughing exercises

    c. Collection of moisture in the oxygen tubing that creates a bubbling sound

    d. Audible gurgling sounds when the client breathes

© 2011 Cengage Learning. All Rights Reserved. May not be scanned, copied or duplicated, or posted to a publicly accessible website, in whole or in part.

11. A common nursing diagnosis for a postoperative client is *Risk for ineffective airway clearance.* Which intervention would *not* be appropriate for a client with this potential problem?

    a. Restricting fluid intake

    b. Splinting incision during respiratory hygiene measures

    c. Chest physiotherapy every 2–4 hours

    d. Incentive spirometer every 1–2 hours

12. A common cause of impaired gas exchange when there is evidence of alveolar collapse is called

    _____.

13. What is the maximum time suction should be applied to the respiratory mucosa?

    a. 3–5 seconds

    b. 6–9 seconds

    c. 10–15 seconds

    d. 16–20 seconds

14. Which instruction would be included in the nurse's discharge teaching plan about lifestyle changes that affect oxygenation?

    a. Allergens can be eliminated with air filters.

    b. Long-term use of alcohol improves oxygenation.

    c. Dependence on nicotine can be decreased by joining a smoking cessation program.

    d. Transdermal patches are not effective in reducing nicotine dependence long term.

15. What is the appropriate amount of suction to use when performing oropharyngeal suctioning?

    a. 20–40 mm Hg

    b. 40–60 mm Hg

    c. 60–80 mm Hg

    d. 80–100 mm Hg

16. The nurse suspects a client has a pulmonary bacterial infection because the client's sputum color is

    a. yellow green.

    b. rusty.

    c. black.

    d. pink.

© 2011 Cengage Learning. All Rights Reserved. May not be scanned, copied or duplicated, or posted to a publicly accessible website, in whole or in part.

17. A type of technique that is useful to raise pulmonary secretions and is characterized by short, forceful exhalations prior to actually coughing is called _____.

18. A client is diagnosed with widespread atelectasis because of oxygen toxicity. The nurse realizes this client is experiencing

    a. pneumonia.

    b. collapsed lung.

    c. hemothorax.

    d. adult respiratory distress syndrome.

19. A client with respiratory and cardiac problems is prescribed an ACE inhibitor. The nurse realizes this medication will

    a. affect renal tubules.

    b. lower blood pressure and decrease the workload of the heart.

    c. slow the heart rate.

    d. dilate the coronary arteries.

20. A client tells the nurse that he uses an herb to help promote the loosening of lung secretions. Which herb has this property?

    a. Broom

    b. Thyme

    c. Licorice

    d. Yarrow

Critical Thinking

21. Explain how to maintain the placement of an endotracheal tube in a client who is agitated.

22. A client with a portable home oxygen unit tells the nurse that he turns off the oxygen when his wife wants to smoke a cigarette. Explain how the nurse should instruct this client.

© 2011 Cengage Learning. All Rights Reserved. May not be scanned, copied or duplicated, or posted to a publicly accessible website, in whole or in part.

Activities

23. Become familiar with a variety of oxygen masks, pulse oximeters, chest tubes, endotracheal tubes, and tracheostomy tubes either in the classroom or laboratory setting. Practice changing the ties on the tracheostomy tube. Practice using the pulse oximeter.

24. Contact the local Center for Emergency Medicine, and schedule a time when the class can be instructed in cardiopulmonary resuscitation.

© 2011 Cengage Learning. All Rights Reserved. May not be scanned, copied or duplicated, or posted to a publicly accessible website, in whole or in part.

Chapter 33 Fluids and Electrolytes

1. Match the term in the left column with its definition from the right column.

   _____ solute

   _____ solvent

   _____ electrolyte

   _____ body fluid

   a. The liquid that contains a substance in solution

   b. The substance that dissociates into ions when dissolved

   c. A solution that contains both electrolytes and water

   d. The substance dissolved in a solution

2. Which of the following is the most frequently occurring intracellular cation?

   a. Na^+

   b. K^+

   c. Ca^{++}

   d. Mg^{++}

3. A function of the electrolyte sodium in the body is to

   a. provide strength and durability to the bones and teeth.

   b. regulate vascular osmotic pressure.

   c. regulate the osmolarity of intracellular fluid.

   d. activate enzyme systems within the body.

4. The force that presses outward against a blood vessel wall is

   a. colloid osmotic pressure.

   b. hydrostatic pressure.

   c. osmotic pressure.

   d. the rate of blood flow.

© 2011 Cengage Learning. All Rights Reserved. May not be scanned, copied or duplicated, or posted to a publicly accessible website, in whole or in part.

5. Which statements are true regarding fluid balance? (Select all that apply.)

    a. Overbreathing can increase fluid loss through the lungs.

    b. The lungs normally cause a daily fluid gain of 400 cc.

    c. The kidneys conserve and excrete body water.

    d. The amount of water lost through the skin is consistently small.

6. To determine if acidosis or alkalosis is present, the nurse could *initially* check

    a. pH.

    b. HCO_3.

    c. $Paco_2$.

    d. Base excess.

7. Which disturbance can cause a client to retain fluid and develop low sodium levels?

    a. Low water intakes

    b. SIADH

    c. Renal dysfunction

    d. Diabetes insipidus

8. A client is demonstrating hypoactive bowel sounds, muscle weakness, and tachycardia. The EKG shows an inverted T wave. Which electrolyte imbalance do these assessment findings suggest to the nurse?

    a. Hypokalemia

    b. Hyperkalemia

    c. Hypocalcemia

    d. Hypermagnesemia

9. A client recovering from a thyroidectomy is to be assessed daily for Chvostek's sign. What does a positive sign indicate?

    a. Hypocalcemia

    b. Hypercalcemia

    c. Hypokalemia

    d. Hyperphosphatemia

© 2011 Cengage Learning. All Rights Reserved. May not be scanned, copied or duplicated, or posted to a publicly accessible website, in whole or in part.

10. What should be assessed first if a client is suspected of having an acid-base imbalance?

    a. Arterial blood gases

    b. Hemoglobin and hematocrit

    c. Serum potassium

    d. Serum sodium

11. A client has a high blood pH, normal oxygen, and normal carbon dioxide but an elevated base excess level. These findings indicate

    a. metabolic alkalosis.

    b. metabolic acidosis.

    c. respiratory acidosis.

    d. respiratory alkalosis.

12. How would the nurse document that a client has a moderate amount of edema?

    a. +0

    b. +1

    c. +2

    d. +3

13. The osmolarity of the intravenous solution of dextrose 5% in 0.45% normal saline is

    a. hypotonic.

    b. isotonic.

    c. hypertonic.

14. Which body area will the nurse use to assess an adult client's skin turgor?

    a. Abdomen

    b. Forearm

    c. Hand

    d. Sternum

© 2011 Cengage Learning. All Rights Reserved. May not be scanned, copied or duplicated, or posted to a publicly accessible website, in whole or in part.

15. The nurse assesses a client's laboratory values and determines that the client is overhydrated. The laboratory test that provides this information is the

    a. hematocrit.

    b. hemoglobin.

    c. arterial blood gas.

    d. prothrombin time.

16. Which assessment most accurately determines a client's fluid status?

    a. Daily weights

    b. 24-hour intake and output calculations

    c. Assessment of vital signs every 8 hours

    d. Hemoglobin level

17. The nurse is providing mouth care to a client who is NPO. What should the nurse use to provide this care?

    a. Alcohol mouthwash

    b. Toothpaste and water

    c. Glycerin swabs

    d. Mild soap and water solution

18. The client is receiving 5% dextrose and water with 20 mEq potassium chloride and is complaining of pain at the IV site. The nurse assesses redness, edema, and tenderness. Which action is the most appropriate?

    a. Stop the IV infusion.

    b. Discontinue the IV and apply a warm compress to the site.

    c. Maintain the IV and apply a warm compress.

    d. Discontinue the IV and call the IV infusion nurse.

19. The prescribing practitioner's order reads: 250 cc Normal Saline IV, infuse over 3 hours. The drop factor of the macrotubing is 15 gtt/mL. How many drops per minute will this gravity flow IV infuse?

    a. 15

    b. 21

    c. 40

    d. 83

© 2011 Cengage Learning. All Rights Reserved. May not be scanned, copied or duplicated, or posted to a publicly accessible website, in whole or in part.

20. A client has a primary IV infusing at 125 cc per hour and is prescribed ampicillin 250 mg to be infused in 50 cc of normal saline over 30 minutes. At which rate should the ampicillin be infused?

    a. 50 cc per hour

    b. 100 cc per hour

    c. 150 cc per hour

    d. 200 cc per hour

21. A client is complaining of a tender intravenous infusion site. Upon assessment, the sight is slightly pink, is swollen, and feels warm 2 inches around the infusion site. What do these findings indicate?

    a. Phlebitis

    b. Infiltration

    c. Edema

    d. Thrombus

22. Blood should be infused within 4 hours after initiating the transfusion. Which of the following statements best explains the rationale for the 4-hour limit?

    a. It elevates the hemoglobin and hematocrit levels.

    b. It provides for the client's comfort.

    c. It reduces the risk for the development of hyperkalemia.

    d. It minimizes the risk for the development of a transfusion reaction.

23. Which solution is appropriate to hang as a secondary bag of fluid to flush tubing that will deliver blood?

    a. Normal saline, 0.9%

    b. Ringer's lactate

    c. 0.45% saline

    d. Dextrose 5% in 0.45% saline

24. The nurse has applied povidone-iodine to a client's skin in preparation to insert an intravenous access device. How should the nurse use this preparation on the client's skin?

    a. Apply alcohol over the iodine.

    b. Apply aqueous chlorhexidine over the iodine.

    c. Wipe off the iodine with a sterile gauze pad.

    d. Allow the iodine to air dry completely.

© 2011 Cengage Learning. All Rights Reserved. May not be scanned, copied or duplicated, or posted to a publicly accessible website, in whole or in part.

25. The nurse assesses a large amount of air in the primary tubing of a client's infusing IV. How should the nurse remove this air?

    a. Insert a syringe with needle into a port below the air, and allow the air to enter the syringe as it flows to the client.

    b. Detach the tubing from the needle, and open the clamp to allow fluid to clear the air out of the tubing.

    c. Change the tubing.

    d. Do nothing.

26. Which of the following solutions does the Intravenous Nurses Society recommend to flush an intravenous cannula?

    a. Heparin

    b. Saline

    c. Dextrose 5% and water

    d. 0.5% normal saline and water

27. Which site is the first choice when starting an IV on a client?

    a. Dorsal plexus vein

    b. Median cubital vein

    c. Great saphenous vein

    d. Dorsal metacarpal vein

28. Why should clean gloves be worn when discontinuing an IV?

    a. The client and family expect this. It promotes psychological well-being.

    b. You minimize potential exposure to body fluids.

    c. You reduce the possibility of introducing microorganisms into the open IV insertion site.

29. Which nursing diagnosis would be appropriate for a client who has an IV infusing at KVO rate?

    a. *Fluid volume deficit*

    b. *Risk for infection*

    c. *Altered oral mucous membranes*

    d. *Impaired skin integrity*

© 2011 Cengage Learning. All Rights Reserved. May not be scanned, copied or duplicated, or posted to a publicly accessible website, in whole or in part.

30. The nurse suspects a client is experiencing a transfusion reaction. Place the responses in the correct order.

   _____ a. Notify the health care practitioner.

   _____ b. Obtain a urine specimen and notify the blood bank.

   _____ c. Discontinue the transfusion and tubing.

   _____ d. Replace the infusion with 0.9% sodium chloride.

Critical Thinking

31. Discuss how the body regulates acid-base balance.

32. Explain the elements of the health history that are specific to fluid balance.

Activities

33. Practice selecting appropriate sites for the placement of an intravenous device for a client. Utilize an intravenous placement training arm/device to practice. Alternatively, nurses specifically trained in intravenous access can be invited to the classroom to discuss and demonstrate the insertion of intravenous access devices.

34. Practice preparing intravenous fluids for infusion. To do this, the following equipment is needed: intravenous solutions, time tapes, tubing sets, and sets of orders. Calculate the drip rates for each intravenous order according to the infusion set used.

35. Practice working with intravenous infusion pumps and flow rate regulators. Have a variety of infusion pumps and flow regulators available for the class to use.

© 2011 Cengage Learning. All Rights Reserved. May not be scanned, copied or duplicated, or posted to a publicly accessible website, in whole or in part.

Chapter 34 Nutrition

1. Which of the following is an inorganic nutrient?

    a. Water

    b. Vitamin

    c. Carbohydrate

    d. Protein

2. In a healthy adult, what percentage of total body weight is water?

    a. 20%–30%

    b. 40%–50%

    c. 50%–60%

    d. 60%–70%

3. Which nutrient does pancreatic lipase act on in the digestive process?

    a. Carbohydrate

    b. Protein

    c. Vitamin

    d. Fat

4. Which mineral plays a role in the formation of thyroid hormone?

    a. Iodine

    b. Iron

    c. Copper

    d. Zinc

© 2011 Cengage Learning. All Rights Reserved. May not be scanned, copied or duplicated, or posted to a publicly accessible website, in whole or in part.

5. A client tells the nurse that she does not understand why she is ill since she takes high doses of vitamins every day so that she will not get sick. How should the nurse respond to this client?

   a. "Maybe you are taking the wrong vitamins."

   b. "Maybe you are not taking enough vitamins."

   c. "Maybe you should be taking different vitamins."

   d. "Maybe you are taking too many vitamins."

6. Match the vitamin in the left column with its function from the right column.

   _____ vitamin A   a. Prevents oxidation of polyunsaturated fatty acids

   _____ vitamin D   b. Promotes the metabolism of carbohydrates

   _____ vitamin E   c. Promotes the oxidation of carbohydrates, fats, and protein

   _____ vitamin K   d. Is a coenzyme to protein and carbohydrate metabolism

   _____ vitamin C   e. Supports retinal pigmentation

   _____ vitamin B_1 f. Supports the production of collagen

   _____ vitamin B_2 g. Plays a role in blood clotting

   _____ vitamin B_6 h. Promotes bone and tooth development

7. During the interview, your client states that she read in the newspaper that antioxidants are good for you. She asks, "Which vitamins can I take that have these antioxidants in them?" Which is the correct response?

   a. Vitamins A, C, and E

   b. Vitamin B complex

   c. Vitamins D and K

8. Excess glucose in the body is stored as glycogen in the

   a. liver and muscles.

   b. liver and pancreas.

   c. muscles and brain.

   d. fatty tissue and muscles.

© 2011 Cengage Learning. All Rights Reserved. May not be scanned, copied or duplicated, or posted to a publicly accessible website, in whole or in part.

9. If the body does not have enough carbohydrates, it begins to break down body proteins in order to produce energy. What is the minimum level of carbohydrate ingestion necessary to prevent protein breakdown?

   a.   25–50 grams

   b.   50–100 grams

   c.   100–150 grams

   d.   150–200 grams

10. What is the minimum amount of protein a person must ingest to prevent obligatory protein loss?

   a.   5–10 grams

   b.   10–20 grams

   c.   20–30 grams

   d.   30–40 grams

11. The fat nutrient responsible for the formation of atherosclerosis is

   a.   low-density lipoprotein.

   b.   triglycerides.

   c.   phospholipids.

   d.   cholesterol.

12. A client from another culture tells the nurse that she has worked very hard to achieve her current weight, which is considered obese according to the BMI index. What does this information suggest to the nurse?

   a.   The client has been eating the wrong foods.

   b.   The client is not aware of U.S. standards for weight control.

   c.   The client's culture places a high value on excess weight.

   d.   The client needs to be on a weight reduction eating plan immediately.

13. Using the components listed, build the U.S. food pyramid from left to right with the numbers 1 through 4.

   _____   Fats and oils

   _____   Vegetables and fruits

   _____   Bread, cereal, grains, rice, pasta

   _____   Dairy products and meats

© 2011 Cengage Learning. All Rights Reserved. May not be scanned, copied or duplicated, or posted to a publicly accessible website, in whole or in part.

14. Which assessment finding indicates a protein deficiency?

    a. Headache

    b. Ascites

    c. Gingivitis

    d. Dental caries

15. Which diagnostic test provides a more accurate picture of a client's protein status?

    a. Hemoglobin level

    b. Nitrogen balance

    c. Serum albumin

    d. Prealbumin

16. A client has an increased BUN level and a decreased urine creatinine level. What do these data suggest to the nurse?

    a. Overhydration

    b. Obesity

    c. Vitamin deficiency

    d. Malnutrition

17. What percentage of hospitalized clients is at risk for malnutrition?

    a. 80%

    b. 65%

    c. 40%

    d. 10%

18. Which assessment would indicate to a nurse that the client's diet could be progressed from a clear liquid to a full liquid diet? The client

    a. has hypoactive bowel sounds.

    b. has normal bowel sounds.

    c. reports nausea.

    d. is experiencing severe diarrhea.

© 2011 Cengage Learning. All Rights Reserved. May not be scanned, copied or duplicated, or posted to a publicly accessible website, in whole or in part.

19. Which reflects a diet moderately restricted in sodium?

    a. 2000 mg

    b. 1000 mg

    c. 500 mg

    d. 250 mg

20. Which client would be a candidate for parenteral nutrition? A client who

    a. can only swallow thickened liquids

    b. chokes when attempting to swallow foods or liquids

    c. is experiencing an intestinal obstruction

    d. consistently ingests 25% of food that is served

21. Which action is the proper method to confirm placement of a small-bore feeding tube?

    a. Aspirate gastric contents with a Luer-Lok syringe and check the pH of the contents.

    b. Begin tube feeding that has been tinted with blue food coloring.

    c. Assess breath sounds.

    d. Assess abdominal sounds.

22. Match the diet type with the client problem.

    _____ clear liquid   a. Surgical clients

    _____ mechanical soft   b. Dysphasia

    _____ low-residue   c. Difficulty chewing

    _____ high-fiber   d. Diverticulosis

    _____ fat-controlled   e. Diverticulitis

    _____ candidiases   f. Obesity

    _____ pureed   g. *Candida albicans*

23. A client ordered intermittent bolus tube feedings every 4 hours has a gastric aspirate residual of 200 cc. What should the nurse do?

    a. Hold the tube feeding until the residual diminishes.

    b. Place the client in low Fowler's position.

    c. Administer the bolus tube feeding.

    d. Administer the tube feeding continuously via pump.

© 2011 Cengage Learning. All Rights Reserved. May not be scanned, copied or duplicated, or posted to a publicly accessible website, in whole or in part.

24. Match the following BMI with the CDC classification.

    _____ underweight   a. BMI = 34

    _____ normal   b. BMI = 28

    _____ overweight   c. BMI = 22

    _____ obese   d. BMI = 16

25. List three categories of contributing factors to the nursing diagnosis *Imbalanced nutrition.*

    a. _____

    b. _____

    c. _____

Critical Thinking

26. Explain the nutritional deficiencies that a client might experience if several feet of the jejunum were removed because of disease.

27. Explain refeeding syndrome.

Activities

28. Conduct an individual 3-day food diary. For 3 days, write down everything you eat, including ounces of fluids and solid foods. Invite a nutritionist or dietitian to the classroom to discuss the information documented in the diary. Work with the nutritionist or dietitian to analyze the contents eaten over 3 days, and determine if there are any nutrients out of balance. If you are unable to locate dietitians or nutritionists, access the Web site http://www.mypyramid.gov, and click on Menu Planner, listed in the left-hand column under Interactive Tools. This is an interactive guide that will ask for basic height and weight information. Then, items ingested can be entered into the tool, which will calculate the number of calories and nutrients ingested. Creating a user ID and password will ensure that any menus planned can be accessed again at a later time.

29. Have a variety of calipers and measuring devices available. Practice using these measuring devices.

30. Have a variety of enteral tubes available. Practice using these tubes for continuous infusion, bolus infusion, and assessing responses to feedings.

31. Using the Internet, research disorders of malabsorption (such as sprue or lactose intolerance), and review the types of eating plans suggested. Study the eating plans to determine if nutrient imbalances can occur, and suggest what can be done to alleviate the imbalances. Discuss the information in small groups.

© 2011 Cengage Learning. All Rights Reserved. May not be scanned, copied or duplicated, or posted to a publicly accessible website, in whole or in part.

Chapter 35 Comfort and Sleep

1. Pain is a _____ experience that is difficult to describe.

2. Which describes pain originating in the internal organs?

    a. Visceral pain

    b. Somatic pain

    c. Cutaneous pain

    d. Neuralgia

3. The changing of noxious stimuli in sensory nerve endings to energy impulses is referred to as

    a. modulation.

    b. transduction.

    c. transmission.

    d. perception.

4. The four vital signs are blood pressure, temperature, pulse, and respiration. Which is now considered the "fifth" vital sign?

    a. Comfort

    b. Sleep

    c. Hydration status

    d. Pain level

5. For which type of pain would oxygen administration be indicated?

    a. Colic

    b. Ischemic

    c. Neuropathic

    d. Myofascial

© 2011 Cengage Learning. All Rights Reserved. May not be scanned, copied or duplicated, or posted to a publicly accessible website, in whole or in part.

6. While assessing a client's amount of pain, the nurse asks, "What makes the pain worse?" Which characteristic of the client's pain is the nurse assessing?

   a. Quality

   b. Intensity

   c. Duration

   d. Triggers

7. Which nursing intervention has a basis in the gate control theory of pain management?

   a. Administering acetaminophen (Tylenol) as ordered

   b. Distracting the client with television

   c. Administering a back massage

   d. Allowing the client to express negative feelings

8. The nurse needs to assess a 2-year-old client for pain. Which scale can the nurse use to help with this assessment?

   a. Wong-Baker Faces Rating Scale

   b. Verbal rating scale

   c. Numeric rating scale

   d. Scream rating scale

9. A client tells the nurse that she has had arthritic pain for years, has difficulty ambulating, and has gained 10 lb over the past 2 months. The most appropriate nursing diagnosis for this client is

   a. *Pain.*

   b. *Chronic pain.*

   c. *Acute pain.*

   d. *Fatigue.*

10. What is the major advantage of using a PCA pump in pain management?

   a. The pharmacy prepares the medication.

   b. It is possible to administer more than the usual and customary dose of an analgesic.

   c. The pain management team is responsible for accuracy of the dose prescription.

   d. The client can control the dosing of the analgesic.

© 2011 Cengage Learning. All Rights Reserved. May not be scanned, copied or duplicated, or posted to a publicly accessible website, in whole or in part.

11. Match the pain intervention in the left column with its definition from the right column.

_____ distraction

_____ imagery

_____ biofeedback

_____ progressive
           muscle relaxation

_____ TENS

a. Focuses the attention away from the pain

b. Helps clients learn to influence their physiological responses

c. Applies minute amounts of electrical stimulation to large-diameter nerve fibers

d. Leads to a reduction in skeletal muscle tension

e. Focuses attention on a mental picture

12. A client has neuropathic pain. Which adjuvant medication could help with this client's pain control?

a. Antihistamine

b. Neuroleptic

c. Tricyclic antidepressant

d. Corticosteroid

13. Which is an advantage of using the intravenous versus subcutaneous opioid infusion as a route of medication administration?

a. There is no associated tissue volume restriction.

b. There is less risk for infection to the insertion site.

c. It provides more effective pain relief.

d. It requires pharmacy support in order to deliver the medication.

14. Based on what you know about the "ceiling effect," which statement would you make when educating family members about medicating a child with an analgesic?

a. "If your child's pain is not affected by this medication, it is okay to increase the dose by half."

b. "If your child's pain is not decreased by this medication, stop the medication and call the prescribing practitioner."

c. "If your child's pain is not affected by this medication, do not increase the dose; the effect is the same, but the risk for experiencing side effects increases."

d. "If your child's pain is not decreased by this medication, call the prescribing practitioner for a new medication prescription."

© 2011 Cengage Learning. All Rights Reserved. May not be scanned, copied or duplicated, or posted to a publicly accessible website, in whole or in part.

15. Match the term in the left column with its definition from the right column.

    _____ addiction   a. Results in withdrawal symptoms when drug is stopped suddenly

    _____ tolerance   b. Psychological dependence

    _____ physical   c. Client requires a larger dose of medication to achieve
              dependence   the same effect

16. A 10-year-old client weighs 98 lb and is ordered morphine for pain. The recommended dosing for a child who weighs less than 50 kg is 0.1 mg/kg. What is the safest dose for this client?

    a. 4 mg

    b. 6 mg

    c. 2 mg

    d. 8 mg

17. The nurse is going to anesthetize a client's skin before inserting an intravenous line. The best topical medication for this procedure is

    a. TAC.

    b. EMLA.

    c. capsaicin cream.

    d. lidocaine patch.

18. Match the term in the left column with its definition from the right column.

    _____ narcolepsy   a. Manifests by clients sleeping excessively

    _____ hypersomnia   b. Pauses in breathing of 30–60 seconds during sleep

    _____ sleep apnea   c. Grinding of the teeth during sleep

    _____ sleep deprivation   d. Sleepwalking

    _____ somnambulism   e. Sudden uncontrollable urges to fall asleep during the day

    _____ bruxism   f. Prolonged inadequacy of quality and quantity of sleep

19. An 80-year-old client is admitted to the hospital to rule out a hip fracture. Which nonverbal behavior would indicate the client is in pain?

    a. Crying or moaning

    b. Frowning or grimacing

    c. Increased muscle tension

    d. All of the above

© 2011 Cengage Learning. All Rights Reserved. May not be scanned, copied or duplicated, or posted to a publicly accessible website, in whole or in part.

20.   A client says that she is "old" and "expects to have pain." How should the nurse respond to this client?

   a.   "Pain is not an inevitable part of aging."

   b.   "If you are in pain, we can treat you."

   c.   "Would you please scale your pain for me?"

   d.   "Aging can be painful."

Critical Thinking

21.   Explain the stages of sleep.

22.   Discuss pharmacological interventions for a client with a sleep disturbance.

Activities

23.   Access the Web site http://www.pain.com. Select the CME Center link. Select the first link under Articles, and read the information in the article "Parent/Nurse-Controlled Analgesia (PNCA) as a Standard of Care: How to Make It Safe." Discuss the information from the article in small groups.

24.   Experience a variety of relaxation techniques. Play a progressive relaxation CD in the class, or have an instructor of meditation attend the class and guide students in progressive relaxation, imagery, biofeedback, and other relaxation techniques.

25.   Invite a colleague from a pain control clinic to come to the class and discuss current approaches in pain management. Be prepared with questions about approaches used in the hospital as well as for the client at home. Which types of approaches work better for which types of pain problems?

© 2011 Cengage Learning. All Rights Reserved. May not be scanned, copied or duplicated, or posted to a publicly accessible website, in whole or in part.

Chapter 36 Mobility

1. Nurses are encouraged by their employers to use good body mechanics. What is meant by "good body mechanics"?

   a. Body parts in the proper position in relation to each other, allowing the body to maintain equilibrium

   b. The use of body parts and positions during activity in order to reduce strain

   c. The use of body parts and positions in order to maintain balance

   d. The awareness of posture, movement, and changes in equilibrium in relation to the body

2. Which reflects the effects of immobility on the musculoskeletal system?

   a. Risk of thrombi formation

   b. Protein anabolism

   c. Calcium loss

   d. Increased respiratory capacity

3. Increased dietary protein is provided for clients who are immobile. Which statement best explains the reason for this intervention?

   a. This is an attempt at the prevention of pressure ulcers.

   b. Negative nitrogen balance occurs.

   c. Peristalsis decreases; therefore, clients lose their appetites.

   d. There is a tendency for the immobile to form renal calculi.

4. A client was admitted with the diagnosis of cerebral vascular accident with the right side affected. The client is confused and cannot feed or bathe herself. Based on this information, which nursing diagnosis is most appropriate for the client at this time?

   a. *Self-care deficits*

   b. *Impaired physical mobility*

   c. *Activity intolerance*

   d. *Risk for aspiration*

© 2011 Cengage Learning. All Rights Reserved. May not be scanned, copied or duplicated, or posted to a publicly accessible website, in whole or in part.

5. Which instruction about good body posture should be provided to a client when ambulating?

   a. Stand with your back straight.

   b. Tuck your abdominal muscles in.

   c. Walk with your head up, and face forward.

   d. All of these instructions.

6. Match each term from the left column with its definition from the right column.

   _____ active ROM   a. Bending of the joint so that articulating bones are moved farther apart

   _____ passive ROM   b. One body part being across another body part at least 180 degrees

   _____ adduction   c. ROM performed by the client

   _____ supination   d. ROM performed by the nurse

   _____ opposition   e. Turning the body or body part upward

   _____ extension   f. Moving toward the midline

7. Exercise increases metabolism, resulting in _____.

8. A client's head of bed is to be maintained in high Fowler's position. In which angle position would the nurse place this client?

   a. 30 degrees

   b. 45 degrees

   c. 60 degrees

   d. 75 degrees

9. Which type of exercise would you advise a client with a cardiovascular problem to avoid?

   a. Isometric

   b. Aerobic

   c. Isotonic

   d. Isokinetic

© 2011 Cengage Learning. All Rights Reserved. May not be scanned, copied or duplicated, or posted to a publicly accessible website, in whole or in part.

10. Which misalignment of the spine would you expect to find during an assessment of an elderly female client?

    a. Scoliosis

    b. Lordosis

    c. Kyphosis

11. Which assessment is *not* common to both skeletal and skin traction?

    a. Body position

    b. Traction weights

    c. Traction rope

    d. Appearance of pin or wire site

12. A client care technician asks the nurse how to assist a client with walking when the client has a chest tube. How should the nurse respond?

    a. Disconnect the chest drainage system from the client; put a 4 × 4 gauze dressing over the chest tube and pin it to his gown. Reconnect it when he returns to his room.

    b. Disconnect the drainage system from the wall suction; put the system on a cart, keeping it upright; ambulate him; then rehook it to the suction when he returns to his room.

    c. You can't ambulate him; he has a chest tube in.

    d. I will help you and hold the drainage system while you support him with walking.

13. A condition of fixed resistance to the passive stretch of muscle is _____.

14. The nurse caring for a comatose client asks his wife to bring in high-top tennis shoes. The purpose of these shoes is to

    a. be used when he regains consciousness.

    b. relieve pressure on the heels.

    c. prevent foot drop.

    d. improve circulation to the feet.

15. The maximum number of hours a client should stay in one position is _____.

© 2011 Cengage Learning. All Rights Reserved. May not be scanned, copied or duplicated, or posted to a publicly accessible website, in whole or in part.

16. When lifting an object, bend at the knees, not the waist. What is the principle behind this practice of good body mechanics?

    a. It provides a stable base to lift from.

    b. It is a more comfortable posture.

    c. It provides greater leverage for lifting.

    d. It supports the back muscles.

17. Which crutch gait is used when one leg is non–weight bearing?

    a. Four-point

    b. Three-point

    c. Two-point

    d. Swing-through

18. The following are all factors that, when combined, could place a client at risk for falls. According to the Risk Assessment Tool for Falls, which factor *alone* places the client at risk for a fall?

    a. Urinary frequency

    b. Vision impairment

    c. Confusion

    d. Use of a cane

19. A client recovering from a total hip replacement is to have an abductor pillow in place. What is the purpose of this pillow?

    a. To improve the circulation to the surgical area

    b. To immobilize the hip joint

    c. To ensure that the affected leg does not move laterally

    d. To prevent the right hip from the flexion and extension movement

20. The most appropriate nursing diagnosis for a client recovering from a total hip replacement is

    a. *Activity intolerance* related to weakness and fatigue.

    b. *Impaired physical mobility* related to musculoskeletal impairment.

    c. *Risk for disuse syndrome* related to mechanical immobilization.

    d. *Self-care deficit* related to pain.

© 2011 Cengage Learning. All Rights Reserved. May not be scanned, copied or duplicated, or posted to a publicly accessible website, in whole or in part.

Critical Thinking

21.   Discuss the cardiovascular effects of exercise.

22.   Explain the three concepts that nurses need to be aware of when positioning clients.

Activities

23.   Practice turning, rolling, and positioning by using a variety of equipment and devices. To do these activities correctly, a room should be established that has practice beds, ambulatory assistive devices (walkers, canes, crutches), splints, pillows, foam wedges, trochanter rolls, foot boards, bed boards, wrist/ hand splints, side rails, and restraints.

24.   Practice conducting range-of-motion exercises. Refer to Table 36-4 for the explanation of each exercise.

25.   Practice ambulating. To do this effectively, have a variety of intravenous poles and other devices that can be simulated as complicating the ambulation process.

26.   Invite physical therapists into the classroom to demonstrate a variety of exercises used to assist and improve the mobility status of clients.

© 2011 Cengage Learning. All Rights Reserved. May not be scanned, copied or duplicated, or posted to a publicly accessible website, in whole or in part.

Chapter 37 Skin Integrity and Wound Healing

1. During wound healing, in which phase does collagen deposition occur?

   a. Defensive

   b. Reconstructive

   c. Maturation

   d. Contraction

2. Match the term in the left column with its definition from the right column.

   _____ phagocytosis   a. Includes new blood vessels and connective tissue

   _____ exudates   b. Formation of blood vessels

   _____ granulation tissue   c. Necrotic tissue

   _____ angiogenesis   d. Envelopment and destruction of microorganisms by leukocytes

   _____ hematoma   e. Collection of blood under the skin

   _____ eschar   f. Fluid and other material that accumulates in wounds

3. A postoperative client has thick yellow drainage around the surgical wound edges. The nurse identifies this drainage as

   a. serous.

   b. purulent.

   c. sanguineous.

   d. serosanguineous.

4. Homeostasis and inflammation are phases of _____.

© 2011 Cengage Learning. All Rights Reserved. May not be scanned, copied or duplicated, or posted to a publicly accessible website, in whole or in part.

5. A 37-year-old client with a history of diabetes is admitted for the debridement of a leg ulcer that has not healed in 2 months. This client is a nonsmoker and takes blood pressure medication. Which of the following is a factor in the client's delayed wound healing?

    a. Age

    b. Blood pressure medication

    c. Diabetes

    d. Nutritional status

6. Skin loss that is confined to epidermal tissue is called a

    a. first-degree wound.

    b. second-degree wound.

    c. third-degree wound.

    d. partial-thickness wound.

7. A client recovering from abdominal surgery tells the nurse that "something popped" when he turned in bed. The nurse assesses the wound and finds that it has eviscerated. What should the nurse do first?

    a. Call his surgeon and the OR.

    b. Apply a dry sterile dressing.

    c. Apply a sterile, saline-soaked dressing.

    d. Apply pressure using a sterile dressing.

8. A client is admitted with a second-degree burn to the left forearm. Which characteristics would the nurse assess about the wound's appearance?

    a. Red and dry

    b. Red and blistery with swelling and exudate

    c. Red and crusty with some blackened areas

9. Which type of drainage system is a Hemovac drain an example of?

    a. Closed suction

    b. Open gravity

    c. Open suction

    d. Closed gravity

© 2011 Cengage Learning. All Rights Reserved. May not be scanned, copied or duplicated, or posted to a publicly accessible website, in whole or in part.

10. Which laboratory value would indicate the amount of protein reserves available for wound healing?

    a. Albumin

    b. WBC

    c. RBC

    d. Cholesterol

11. For which client would a nurse be on the alert for a risk for injury when applying a hot pack?

    a. A 5-year-old with an infection under the fingernail

    b. A 45-year-old cardiac-diseased client with an IV infiltrate

    c. An 80-year-old client with diabetes and with a wound infection

12. A 4-year-old client comes to the emergency department with a head laceration. The wound is bleeding profusely, and the client is in pain. The wound is cleansed and covered with a sterile gauze dressing. What should be placed over the dressing?

    a. An Aqua K pad (aquathermia unit)

    b. A warm washcloth

    c. An ice bag

    d. A cold, wet compress

13. List three nursing diagnoses that address the client's psychological responses to changes in skin integrity.

    a. _____

    b. _____

    c. _____

14. Which irrigation solution would be most appropriate for cleansing an infected wound?

    a. Full-strength hydrogen peroxide

    b. Full-strength Provo-iodine

    c. Sterile saline

    d. Half-strength hydrogen peroxide

© 2011 Cengage Learning. All Rights Reserved. May not be scanned, copied or duplicated, or posted to a publicly accessible website, in whole or in part.

15. A client is recovering from the debridement of an infected sternal wound after coronary artery bypass surgery. The wound is open and is to have wet-to-dry saline dressing changes four times a day. Which type of wound healing is this considered?

    a. Primary intention healing

    b. Secondary intention healing

    c. Tertiary intention healing

16. Which intervention would be appropriate on a nursing care plan when a client is at high risk for skin breakdown?

    a. Massage bony prominences four times a day.

    b. Use alcohol during back rubs; perform three times a day.

    c. Turn and reposition every 2 hours.

    d. Place a donut on the wheelchair seat while client is up in the wheelchair.

17. Which type of dressings would be used for a stage II pressure ulcer with moderate amounts of drainage?

    a. Transparent adhesive (e.g., Tegaderm)

    b. Hydrogel (e.g., Carrasyn Hydrogel Wound Dressing)

    c. Exudate absorber (e.g., Debrisan)

    d. Hydrocolloid (e.g., DuoDERM)

18. A warm compress will be applied to the site of an infiltrated intravenous line. How long should this compress be applied?

    a. 10 minutes

    b. 20 minutes

    c. 40 minutes

    d. 60 minutes

19. An assessment of the client's nutritional status should evaluate

    a. albumin level.

    b. prealbumin level.

    c. weight.

    d. nutritional intake.

    e. all of the above.

© 2011 Cengage Learning. All Rights Reserved. May not be scanned, copied or duplicated, or posted to a publicly accessible website, in whole or in part.

20.   Which assessment is a predictor of skin breakdown?

   a.   Stage II pressure ulcer

   b.   Persistent erythema of the skin

   c.   Blanching when pressure is applied to the skin

   d.   Ischemia

Critical Thinking

21.   Describe the stages of pressure ulcers.

22.   Compare the Braden Scale for Predicting Pressure Sore Risk with the Norton Scale for Pressure Ulcer Risk.

Activities

23.   Practice opening, preparing, and applying dressings to a variety of wounds, with and without drains. All of the necessary supplies should be provided in addition to practice wound sites on training arms and other body areas.

24.   Invite nurses and other health care professionals to the class to discuss the care of wounds. If possible, invite nurses who provide burn care. Be prepared with questions to ask the panel of care providers regarding specific challenges, wound care approaches, and other care issues when providing care to the client with burns or other large wounds.

25.   Access the Wound Care Information Network at http://www.medicaledu.com. Scroll through the topics on the left-hand column, and read information under each of the levels of wounds identified. Discuss how this site can serve as a resource when providing wound care to clients.

© 2011 Cengage Learning. All Rights Reserved. May not be scanned, copied or duplicated, or posted to a publicly accessible website, in whole or in part.

Chapter 38 Sensation, Perception, and Cognition

1. Which part of the brain is responsible for maintaining equilibrium?

   a. Cerebrum

   b. Brain stem

   c. Cerebellum

   d. Broca's area

2. An individual is said to have fluid intelligence when he or she demonstrates

   a. conceptual understanding.

   b. adaptability.

   c. cognitive flow states.

   d. memory impairment.

3. Which of the following controls sleep/wakefulness and consciousness?

   a. The glossopharyngeal nerve

   b. The somatic nervous system

   c. The diencephalon

   d. The reticular activating system

4. A client states, "The president of the United States is telling me that I must leave this place." This statement is an example of

   a. an illusion.

   b. a visual hallucination.

   c. an auditory hallucination.

   d. poor judgment.

© 2011 Cengage Learning. All Rights Reserved. May not be scanned, copied or duplicated, or posted to a publicly accessible website, in whole or in part.

5. Which situation would place a client at risk for developing sensory overload?

    a. A 10-year-old in the x-ray department waiting for a chest x-ray

    b. A 79-year-old in the intensive care unit recovering from surgery

    c. A 40-year-old, with a chief complaint of a skin rash, being evaluated by a nurse practitioner

    d. An 85-year-old receiving a vitamin injection in her home by a visiting nurse

6. A 90-year-old female client is hard of hearing, cannot ambulate, and speaks only Italian. The family members tell the nurse that the client is lonely because most of her friends have died and the family cannot visit as much as they would like. Which nursing diagnosis would be appropriate for the client at this time?

    a. *Social isolation*

    b. *Altered thought process*

    c. *Sensory-perceptual alteration: hearing*

    d. *Ineffective family coping*

7. A client is able to tell the nurse his name but not the day or where he is located. He does know that he has been ill but cannot recall the reason for the hospitalization. The nurse should document this client's orientation as

    a. oriented × 1.

    b. oriented × 2.

    c. oriented × 3.

8. An effective method of reorienting clients would be to

    a. state their name and their room number.

    b. state their name, the day, and time.

    c. state their name and when lunch will be served.

9. A client's level of consciousness has changed from alert to obtunded. Which characteristics will the nurse assess in this client?

    a. Nonverbal, unable to follow commands, but does move if stimulated

    b. Unconscious with no meaningful response to stimuli

    c. Slow to respond, drifts off to sleep when not stimulated

    d. Sleeps most of the time, inconsistently follows commands, difficult to arouse

© 2011 Cengage Learning. All Rights Reserved. May not be scanned, copied or duplicated, or posted to a publicly accessible website, in whole or in part.

10. What instructions should the nurse give to a client experiencing a tactile deficit?

    a. Use assistive devices such as a hearing aid.

    b. Place a calendar and clock in rooms that you frequent.

    c. Avoid using heating pads.

    d. Purchase books on tape or books that contain large print.

11. Which client would be able to independently take a shower?

    a. Alert and oriented client

    b. Confused client

    c. Client who is hallucinating

    d. Client who is lethargic

12. Which action should be included when caring for an unconscious client?

    a. Keep the bed at the level most comfortable for the nurse to provide care.

    b. Explain all procedures.

    c. Keep the room quiet.

    d. Limit conversation and visitors.

13. A client has the nursing diagnosis of *Disturbed thought processes*. Which intervention should be included in this client's plan of care?

    a. Keep the environment calm.

    b. Monitor client closely; check every 30 minutes.

    c. Use physical restraints prn.

    d. Participate in large-group activities as often as possible.

14. Which nursing diagnosis is a priority for a client who is experiencing an altered level of consciousness?

    a. *Disturbed sensory perception*

    b. *Risk for injury*

    c. *Disturbed thought processes*

    d. *Disturbed body image*

© 2011 Cengage Learning. All Rights Reserved. May not be scanned, copied or duplicated, or posted to a publicly accessible website, in whole or in part.

15. Which intervention would be appropriate for a client experiencing a visual impairment?

   a. Use brief, concise statements.

   b. Speak in raised tones.

   c. Keep objects in their usual place.

   d. Provide a private room whenever possible.

16. Long-term exposure to loud sounds may result in

   a. a tension headache.

   b. anxiety.

   c. hypertension.

   d. all of the above.

17. A client cannot remember if she had any visitors yesterday but can clearly recall events from her early adulthood. This client's memory would be considered as having

   a. recent recall but poor long-term memory.

   b. intact long-term memory but limited recent recall.

   c. intact long-term memory but poor immediate memory.

18. A commonly used nursing intervention is client teaching. Which statement best supports the strategy to delay client teaching when a client's anxiety level is high?

   a. As the anxiety level increases, it interferes with the client's ability to concentrate by decreasing his or her attention span.

   b. During high-anxiety periods, efferent nerve pathways are stimulated, which causes a disruption in memory.

   c. Anxiety interferes with the brain's ability to interpret speech.

   d. Anxiety causes the reticular activating system to misfire, leading to a change in level of consciousness.

19. It is documented that a client has "poor impulse control." Which component of cognition was assessed for this client?

   a. Affect

   b. Judgment

   c. Perception

   d. Memory

© 2011 Cengage Learning. All Rights Reserved. May not be scanned, copied or duplicated, or posted to a publicly accessible website, in whole or in part.

20. Which medication would *not* contribute to the alteration in level of consciousness?

    a.   Morphine sulfate (analgesic)

    b.   Librium (benzodiazepine)

    c.   Phenobarbital (sedative)

    d.   Insulin (antidiabetic agent)

Critical Thinking

21. Explain the components of the Glasgow Coma Scale.

22. Discuss the role of herbal therapy in the central nervous system.

Activities

23. Create a mnemonic to recall the cranial nerves. (For example, Oh oh oh the train abounds far! Very good vision, says Helen!)

24. Practice assessing the cranial nerves. Have available cotton swabs, tongue blades, pen lights, and other devices to successfully assess each cranial nerve.

25. Experience sensory deficits. To do this, have available ear muffs or ear plugs, eyewear covered with waxed paper or coated with petroleum jelly, and heavy gloves or other padding. Take turns using each item to simulate visual, hearing, and tactile deficits. Attempt to participate in conversations, see what others are doing, and pick up common items in the environment such as a pen or pencil, piece of paper, or container of fluid. Discuss the challenges associated with using each item that altered the hearing, vision, or tactile perception. How will this experience help when providing care to clients with these types of sensory deficits?

© 2011 Cengage Learning. All Rights Reserved. May not be scanned, copied or duplicated, or posted to a publicly accessible website, in whole or in part.

Chapter 39 Elimination

1. Match the term in the left column with its definition in the right column.

   _____ incontinence   a. Progressive rhythmic muscle contraction

   _____ peristalsis   b. Pus in the urine

   _____ defecation   c. Painful or difficult urination

   _____ flatulence   d. Bacteria in the urine

   _____ pyuria   e. Uncontrolled loss of urine or stool

   _____ bacteriuria   f. Evacuation of stool from the rectum

   _____ dysuria   g. Inability to completely empty the bladder during micturition

   _____ retention   h. Discharge of gas from the rectum

2. Which body structure varies significantly between men and women?

   a. Urethra

   b. Ureter

   c. Bladder

   d. Sigmoid colon

3. Which muscle allows adults to postpone urination?

   a. Detrusor

   b. Urogenital diaphragm

   c. Valves of Houston

   d. Depressor

4. Which condition, if left uncorrected, can lead to urinary retention?

   a. Benign prostatic hypertrophy

   b. Diabetes

   c. Multiple sclerosis

   d. Cystitis

© 2011 Cengage Learning. All Rights Reserved. May not be scanned, copied or duplicated, or posted to a publicly accessible website, in whole or in part.

5. Which food promotes constipation?

   a. Cheese

   b. Chocolate

   c. Celery

   d. Popcorn

6. A 78-year-old client is becoming increasingly disoriented and anxious. The client is unable to hold her urine after recognizing the need to void and is incontinent when ambulating to the bathroom. Which type of incontinence describes what this client is demonstrating?

   a. Functional incontinence

   b. Urge incontinence

   c. Stress incontinence

   d. Total incontinence

7. The laboratory analysis of a client's urine states that red blood cells are present. This finding would be considered

   a. pyuria.

   b. dysuria.

   c. bacteriuria.

   d. hematuria.

8. An increase in intraabdominal pressure along with atrophy of urethral tissue diminishes the urethra's

   _____.

9. Clients receiving enteral feedings can experience diarrhea. Which best explains the reason for this?

   a. Digestion is impaired.

   b. The feedings contain a high osmolality.

   c. The feedings damage the GI mucosa.

   d. Clients who require enteral feedings are experiencing a high catabolic state.

10. Which medication can lead to urinary retention?

    a. Antihypertensive

    b. Insulin

    c. Topical anesthetic

    d. Senna

© 2011 Cengage Learning. All Rights Reserved. May not be scanned, copied or duplicated, or posted to a publicly accessible website, in whole or in part.

11. A client tells the nurse that she takes mineral oil every day to keep her bowels moving regularly. What should the nurse do regarding this information?

    a. Do nothing; mineral oil is a commonly used laxative.

    b. Provide education; mineral oil can interfere with vitamin absorption.

    c. Advise against taking mineral oil; there are less harmful laxatives on the market.

12. The penises of clients who use condom catheters to manage urinary incontinence must be assessed regularly. What is the reason for this?

    a. To check for lesions or rashes

    b. To check for leakage

    c. To check for twisting of the condom catheter

    d. All of the above

13. A client with constipation has very dry, hard stools. Which type of enema would be indicated for this client?

    a. Kayexalate

    b. Oil retention

    c. Carminative

    d. Antibiotic

14. How would you position a client when preparing to administer an enema?

    a. Left-side lying

    b. Right-side lying

    c. Prone

    d. Semi-Fowler's

15. Which is most likely to be a temporary bowel diversion?

    a. Double-barrel stoma

    b. End stoma

    c. Ileostomy

    d. Sigmoid colostomy

© 2011 Cengage Learning. All Rights Reserved. May not be scanned, copied or duplicated, or posted to a publicly accessible website, in whole or in part.

16. When administering an enema "until clear," the nurse should not exceed _____ liters of fluid in any one series of enemas.

    a. 1.5

    b. 2

    c. 3

    d. 2.5

17. Match each of the foods with the level of fiber content.

    _____ a. milk   1. High fiber

    _____ b. beans   2. Low fiber

    _____ c. white rice

    _____ d. corn

    _____ e. apples

    _____ f. watermelon

    _____ g. acorn squash

18. If a nurse assesses a client's stoma as being dark and dusky, the first action the nurse should do is _____.

19. A client is diagnosed with a *Clostridium difficile* infection. Which symptom is this client most likely demonstrating?

    a. Constipation

    b. Diarrhea

    c. Urge urinary incontinence

    d. Hematuria

20. A client is prescribed Ditropan for urge urinary incontinence. Which instruction should the nurse *not* give to this client?

    a. Decrease the intake of bladder irritants, such as caffeine and high-acid juices.

    b. Adhere to a regular-timed voiding schedule.

    c. Increase fluids rich in electrolytes.

© 2011 Cengage Learning. All Rights Reserved. May not be scanned, copied or duplicated, or posted to a publicly accessible website, in whole or in part.

Critical Thinking

21.   Explain the impact of age on bowel elimination.

22.   How should a middle-aged male client be instructed regarding the risk of intrinsic sphincter deficiency after a radical prostatectomy?

Activities

23.   Practice preparing to administer an enema to a client. To do this, all equipment should be available for use.

24.   Practice catheterizing a male and female client. Ensure that different catheterization sizes are available as well as a training torso designed for catheterization practice.

25.   Access the Wound, Ostomy and Continence Nurses Society Web site at http://www.wocn.org. Click on the link to the WOCN Library, and then click on White Papers under Accessible in the Library. Read the white paper, and discuss the information learned in small groups or as a full class.

© 2011 Cengage Learning. All Rights Reserved. May not be scanned, copied or duplicated, or posted to a publicly accessible website, in whole or in part.

Chapter 40 Nursing Care of the Perioperative Client

1. In which type of surgical intervention would a surgeon not be able to discuss the setting and scheduling of the client's surgery?

   a. Emergency surgery

   b. Urgent surgery

   c. Elective surgery

2. Match the surgical intervention in the left column with its purpose from the right column.

   _____ diagnostic

   _____ reconstructive

   _____ curative

   _____ palliative

   _____ transplant

   a. Remove diseased tissue or organ and replace it with functioning tissue or organ

   b. Decrease the spread of a disease process to prolong life or to alleviate pain

   c. Repair or remove a diseased organ or restore normal physiological functioning

   d. Determine the origin of presenting symptoms and the extent of a disease process

   e. Correct a disease process or improve a cosmetic appearance

3. Prior to the start of any surgical or invasive procedure, all of the following are Joint Commission National Patient Safety Goal requirements except

   a. conduct a "time out" prior to the procedure.

   b. mark the site of the operation or procedure.

   c. sign the preoperative checklist.

   d. involve the client in the preoperative marking process.

© 2011 Cengage Learning. All Rights Reserved. May not be scanned, copied or duplicated, or posted to a publicly accessible website, in whole or in part.

4. Match the type of anesthesia in the left column with its effects from the right column.

_____ general anesthesia

_____ regional anesthesia

_____ major/minor nerve block

_____ intravenous regional anesthesia

a. Temporary decreased sensation or loss of feeling and movement to the lower part of the body; drug injected through a needle or catheter placed directly into the spinal canal

b. Temporary loss of feeling or movement of an extremity; drug injected into veins of arm or leg

c. Total unconscious state administered through inhalation or injection

d. Temporary loss of feeling or movement to a specific limb or area of the body; drug injected near multiple nerves or plexus

5. During which part of the preoperative assessment will the nurse discuss any anesthesia complications from previous surgeries with the client?

a. Medical history

b. Nursing history

c. Medications

d. Physical assessment

6. A client planning to undergo a surgical procedure is underweight. Which nursing diagnosis does the nurse realize is appropriate for this client?

a. *Anxiety*

b. *Ineffective tissue perfusion*

c. *Acute pain*

d. *Risk for infection*

7. Which is an appropriate nursing intervention after a client has been anesthetized with an oral anesthetic solution such as viscous lidocaine?

a. Rinse the mouth with saline solution until sensation returns.

b. Offer foods of pudding-like consistency until swallowing returns.

c. Keep the client NPO until the gag reflex returns.

d. Do not offer the client hot liquids until sensation returns.

© 2011 Cengage Learning. All Rights Reserved. May not be scanned, copied or duplicated, or posted to a publicly accessible website, in whole or in part.

8. Why should the nurse assess a client's use of herbal remedies prior to undergoing a surgical procedure?

   a. To determine allergies

   b. To determine if the herbs place the client at risk if taken before surgery

   c. To determine if the herb will enhance healing

   d. To determine if the client can cope with missing the herb after surgery

9. Which drug places the client at risk for intra- and postoperative bleeding?

   a. Aspirin (nonnarcotic analgesic, antipyretic)

   b. Prednisone (steroid)

   c. Sominex (bromide in combination)

   d. Amitriptyline (antidepressant)

10. Which of the following statements best explains the reason for performing and documenting the results of a nursing preoperative physical assessment?

    a. It is a requirement of the hospital.

    b. It provides a baseline for comparison of postoperative findings.

    c. It assists the nurse in beginning discharge planning.

    d. It replaces the prescribing practitioner's physical examination in some surgery centers.

11. Match the perioperative phase in the left column with the nursing diagnosis from the right column that is most likely to be relevant to clients within that perioperative phase.

    _____ preoperative   a. *Anxiety* related to risk factors of surgery and anesthesia

    _____ intraoperative   b. *Ineffective airway clearance* related to anesthesia

    _____ postoperative   c. *Risk for injury* related to positioning

12. Which preoperative procedure will most likely not be listed on a preoperative checklist?

    a. Nail polish and make-up removal

    b. Lab work complete and on the chart

    c. Assessment of the client's anxiety level

    d. Addressograph plate and MAR on the chart

© 2011 Cengage Learning. All Rights Reserved. May not be scanned, copied or duplicated, or posted to a publicly accessible website, in whole or in part.

13. What is the purpose of an incentive spirometer?

   a. To facilitate the removal of anesthesia from the system

   b. To enhance circulation

   c. To achieve sustained maximum inspiration

   d. To reduce the need for intravenous fluids

14. A blood clot or air that moves in the circulatory system from its place of origin is called a(n)

   _____.

15. The recommended frequency for removal of antiembolism stockings is

   a. once a day.

   b. twice a day.

   c. three times a day.

   d. twice in 8 hours.

16. For which of the following types of postoperative management equipment would a nurse be concerned about the lockout interval?

   a. TENS unit

   b. PCA pump

   c. ICD pump

   d. CPM machine

17. Match the surgical team member in the left column with the role of that member from the right column.

   _____ anesthetist   a. Obtains the surgical consent

   _____ surgeon   b. Obtains supplies and delivers materials in the operating room

   _____ first assistant   c. Prepares the instrument tray and passes the instruments to the surgeon

   _____ scrub nurse   d. Performs intubation prior to the beginning of surgery

   _____ circulating nurse   e. Helps the surgeon ligate, suction, and suture

© 2011 Cengage Learning. All Rights Reserved. May not be scanned, copied or duplicated, or posted to a publicly accessible website, in whole or in part.

18. The nurse prevents exposure to blood and body fluids during surgery by performing all of the following *except*

    a. using goggles.

    b. changing gloves periodically.

    c. grounding equipment properly.

    d. disposing properly of sharps.

19. Clients are at high risk for injury related to hypothermia during surgery. Which contributes to bodily heat loss?

    a. Anesthetic agents

    b. Exposure of large operative sites

    c. Exposure to a cold operating room

    d. All of the above

20. Which incision would you expect to find on a postoperative client who had a splenectomy (spleen removal)?

    a. Left oblique subcostal

    b. Thoracoabdominal

    c. Lower vertical midline

    d. Upper vertical midline

21. What should the nurse assess first in a client being admitted to the postanesthesia care unit?

    a. Neurologic status

    b. Fluid status

    c. Pain

    d. Airway and respirations

22. Which of the following is an *abnormal* postoperative nursing assessment finding?

    a. Urinary output of less than 30 cc per hour

    b. Pulse oximeter reading of 96%

    c. Absent bowel sounds

    d. Negative Homans' sign

© 2011 Cengage Learning. All Rights Reserved. May not be scanned, copied or duplicated, or posted to a publicly accessible website, in whole or in part.

23. Which best describes the postoperative complication atelectasis?

    a. It is a lower level of oxygen in the blood.

    b. Pulmonary secretions pool, which leads to decreased pulmonary ventilation.

    c. It is caused by a blood clot in the lungs, which results in pulmonary obstruction.

    d. Inflammation of a vein causes pain and discomfort in the lower extremities.

24. What should a postoperative client be able to do at the time of discharge?

    a. Take his or her own vital signs

    b. Relate symptoms to be reported to the prescribing practitioner

    c. Create a 2-week meal plan for a low-cholesterol diet

    d. Change a complex dressing using sterile technique

25. A 2-day post-thyroidectomy client is ambulating and taking fluids; however, the client cannot perform deep breathing and coughing exercises because of incisional pain. Which nursing diagnosis would be appropriate for this client?

    a. *Altered nutrition: less than body requirements*

    b. *Ineffective airway clearance*

    c. *Risk for infection*

    d. *Acute pain*

Critical Thinking

26. Discuss the roles of the scrub nurse and circulating nurse during an operative procedure.

27. Explain the criteria used to determine if a client can be extubated after receiving general anesthesia.

Activities

28. Participate in the preparation of a client for a surgical procedure by observing a nurse conduct a preoperative assessment and complete the surgical checklist.

29. Depending on the facility, observe a surgical procedure. Identify the scrub nurse, circulating nurse, surgical first assistant, surgeon, and anesthesiologist. If others are in the operative suite, determine their roles and functions.

30. Access the Association of periOperative Registered Nurses Web site at http://www.aorn.org. What educational resources are available through this Web site? What issues and initiatives are members of the site currently concerned with? What other information is available on the site? Discuss the impact of this Web site on nurses who provide care to clients undergoing surgical procedures.

© 2011 Cengage Learning. All Rights Reserved. May not be scanned, copied or duplicated, or posted to a publicly accessible website, in whole or in part.

Answer Key

Chapter 1

1. b
2. trained
3. d
4. c
5. d
6. a
7. d
8. d, e, c, f, b, h, a, g
9. a
10. b
11. b, d, c, a
12. b
13. c
14. d
15. a
16. d
17. c
18. b
19. a
20. d

Critical Thinking

21. Nightingale advocated for systematic assessment, individualized care based on needs and preferences, maintaining confidentiality, formally educating nurses, and nurses' role in client advocacy. In addition, she advocated for clean surroundings, including fresh air and light.

22. Today's nurse needs to be prepared to react to a variety of changing conditions. In order to respond appropriately, education must include the care of communities when faced with a natural disaster caused by weather (e.g., tornadoes, hurricanes, tsunamis) or uncontrollable environmental conditions (e.g., wildfires, volcanic eruptions, earthquakes). Because the world is more mobile, diseases that were once restricted are now becoming widespread. Nurses need to be able to respond to these communicable diseases in order to prevent their spread and transmission. The world today is highly volatile. Terrorist groups exist in many nations, and the United States is often a target for the expression of anger by these groups. Terrorism can take many forms, and nurses can participate in the response and rescue by triaging, decontaminating, or becoming members of crisis response units.

Chapter 2

1. c, e, b, f, d, a
2. b
3. b
4. developing nursing practice standards
5. b
6. a
7. d
8. c
9. d
10. b
11. a

© 2011 Cengage Learning. All Rights Reserved. May not be scanned, copied or duplicated, or posted to a publicly accessible website, in whole or in part.

12. a	15. c	18. a
13. d	16. 7, 4, 1, 5, 8, 3, 9, 6, 2	19. a
14. b	17. a	20. a

Critical Thinking

21. Health care in the United States has traditionally been focused on the treatment of disease. Over the last decade, prevention and wellness have been added as health care goals and initiatives. Even though many health care providers still approach client care as the treatment of disease, more recent approaches focus on individual responsibility for health and wellness activities to reduce the likelihood of developing disease in the future. Wellness and prevention initiatives that are surging to the forefront today include weight management, smoking cessation, exercise, stress reduction, routine preventative health care practices, and immunizations for all ages of the life span.

22. The simultaneity paradigm views the person-environment interaction as in unity with the universe. Since the human cannot be separated from the universe, as both change in unpredictable ways, the only way to define health is from an individual client's perspective. The focus of health is on that which the individual defines as "quality of life." A younger person might define quality of life as the ability to work, socialize, marry, raise a family, and enjoy life. An elderly person might define quality of life as being able to perform activities of daily living, live independently, have sufficient financial resources, and not become a burden to society. A person recovering from a motor vehicle accident might define quality of life as the ability to return to work, walk, use an assistive device, or learn to function with the use of a wheelchair. Each person's definition of quality of life is different and will change according to interactions with the environment.

Chapter 3

1. d	7. b	14. c
2. c	8. d	15. c
3. a	9. c	16. d
4. d	10. a	17. c
5. c	11. b	18. d
6. a	12. a	19. b
	13. b, e, d, c, a	20. b

Critical Thinking

21. The nurse has the right to refuse to participate in the study and should do so. The nurse should not feel pressured to participate in research for fear of losing employment or other sanctions.

22. Even though the two terms are often used interchangeably, they have different meanings. Evidence-based practice can be a best practice, but a best practice is not necessarily evidence-based. Best

© 2011 Cengage Learning. All Rights Reserved. May not be scanned, copied or duplicated, or posted to a publicly accessible website, in whole or in part.

practices are ideas and strategies that work to produce positive client outcomes or to reduce costs. Evidence-based practice is the use of the best evidence from research to guide clinical decision making. Evidence-based practice shifts care away from opinion, past practice, and tradition to a more scientific basis.

Chapter 4

1. c

2. b

3. a. Cost
   b. Access
   c. Quality of care

4. b, c, a

5. b, c, a

6. a. Medicare

   b. Medicaid
   c. State Children's Health Insurance Program

7. d

8. c

9. wellness, illness, disability

10. b

11. a

12. d

13. b

14. a

15. a

16. a

17. c

18. d

19. d

20. c

Critical Thinking

21. The client is a consumer or customer of health care services. If an organization is not concerned with the customer's opinion of the services provided, the customer will go to another organization for services, and the health care organization will lose business. Also, the dissatisfied customer will inform others about the services from the facility, which could lead to an additional loss of customers in the future. If a customer is not satisfied with one aspect of the services provided, all additional services from the same health care organization can lose business as well. Because satisfaction is subjective, all health care providers need to listen to the client and value the information provided about customer service.

22. The rising cost of health care is due in part to the age of the population, an increasing number of people with chronic illnesses, technological advances, and too many hospital beds. As the population ages, the need for health care services increases. This factor ties in with an increasing number of people with chronic illnesses. Chronic illnesses increase with age, so if the population is aging, then the incidence of chronic illnesses will also increase. With a chronic illness, the client will not recover; however, he or she can reach a level of maintenance with the illness. There will be periods of exacerbation that will cause the client to seek additional medical services. Also, technology costs money to research, design, develop, create, and distribute. Technological advances have saved many lives and have added to the early diagnosis of health care problems; however, using technology costs money. In addition, because of the access changes to health care, many clients are seeking early intervention through their primary care prescribing practitioners. Some health problems no longer need hospitalization to treat. Fewer clients are being admitted to hospitals, which leads to an overabundance of hospital beds, and each empty bed costs the health care organization money.

© 2011 Cengage Learning. All Rights Reserved. May not be scanned, copied or duplicated, or posted to a publicly accessible website, in whole or in part.

Chapter 5

1. b, c, a

2. critical thinking

3. a

4. d

5. d

6. Habit, Fear of making mistakes, or Use of meaningless routines and rituals

7. a. to identify and classify nursing outcomes
   b. to validate the classification system
   c. to use clinical data to measure outcomes

8. c, a, b, e, d

9. Subjective, Objective, Subjective, Objective, Subjective, Objective

10. d

11. c

12. c

13. b

14. b

15. c

16. d

17. d

18. a

19. b

20. c

Critical Thinking

21. Groupthink is when a person agrees or goes along with the opinion of someone else or others and does not speak up or discuss his or her own differing opinion or belief. The person who engages in groupthink will limit his or her own creative thinking and problem-solving abilities. The person who engages in groupthink might do so in fear of going against the majority or because of not wanting to rock the boat by offering a different opinion. By not speaking up as an individual, a person jeopardizes the critical thinking process, which can limit the problem-solving method.

22. A "risk" nursing diagnosis is when a problem does not yet exist; however, there are risk factors present that could lead to the development of a problem. A "possible" nursing diagnosis is when a problem could occur unless preventive action is taken to avoid the onset of the problem.

Chapter 6

1. c

2. b

3. b

4. a

5. b, a, d, c

6. a. Interview
   b. Health history
   c. Physical examination
   d. Laboratory and diagnostic tests

7. d

8. a. Introduction
   b. Working
   c. Closure

9. d

10. c

11. 6, 3, 2, 1, 5, 4

12. b, a, a, b a

13. a

14. a

15. c

16. c

17. a

18. d

19. a

20. c

© 2011 Cengage Learning. All Rights Reserved. May not be scanned, copied or duplicated, or posted to a publicly accessible website, in whole or in part.

Critical Thinking

21. The body systems model is often referred to as the medical model because the assessment is done according to body systems. When focusing solely on body systems, the client's responses to illness might be overlooked. This model also does not support the client's psychosocial needs. The use of this model contributes to fragmented care.

22. The first thing to do is to find out if someone accompanied the client to the hospital. If so, determine the relationship of the person to the client. Family members or significant others can contribute to the health history, and the nurse should talk with these individuals first. Another thing the nurse can do is access any previous medical records that might exist in the health care organization for the client. The medical records can provide a past medical history, previous health problems, medications prescribed, allergies, and previous functional status. This information can serve as a baseline in the absence of the client's ability to provide it.

Chapter 7

1. a

2. a

3. e

4. a

5. b

6. b

7. *Disuse syndrome, Rape-trauma syndrome,* *Relocation stress syndrome, Sudden infant death syndrome*

8. c

9. c

10. 4, 6, 3 ,7, 1, 2, 5

11. a

12. c

13. a

14. d

15. b

16. b

17. c

18. d

19. domains, classes, diagnostic statements

20. a

Critical Thinking

21. Nurses cannot agree about the NANDA-approved nursing diagnoses list. Areas of disagreement include specific labels used in the classification system and the perception that the list is confining, incomplete, illness and/or disease oriented, and confusing. Some nurses have not received education on how to use the NANDA list or feel that it lacks a diagnosis that is needed for a particular client's problem. Nurses might also hesitate to use a diagnosis of *Noncompliance* or *Knowledge deficit* and would rather not use diagnoses in order to avoid errors in clinical judgment. The use of nursing diagnoses also has legal considerations. If a diagnosis is inappropriate or incomplete, the nurse can be held liable for errors in clinical judgment.

22. The science of nursing continues to evolve, and with that evolution, new ways to describe client problems will be discovered. Nurses should use the current list of approved nursing diagnoses, and when a situation arises that does not fit a diagnosis from the list, efforts should be taken to describe the phenomenon as best as possible. These situations will continue to be submitted to NANDA for further study and consideration to be possibly added to the list of approved diagnoses. Because health care is constantly changing, new client problems will continue to be discovered. There will never be a complete list of nursing diagnoses.

© 2011 Cengage Learning. All Rights Reserved. May not be scanned, copied or duplicated, or posted to a publicly accessible website, in whole or in part.

Chapter 8

1. a. Establishing priorities
   b. Setting goals
   c. Identifying interventions

2. a

3. d, c, b, a, e

4. 1, 3, 4, 2

5. c

6. c

7. d

8. b

9. a

10. b

11. b

12. d

13. a

14. c

15. Detailed description

16. a

17. b

18. a

19. c

20. b

Critical Thinking

21. Ideally, nursing diagnoses should be prioritized from most life threatening to least life threatening. Alternatively, the diagnoses can be prioritized according to high, moderate, and low priority. In the event that the nurse identifies a nursing diagnosis as high priority and the client does not agree, the nurse should discuss the reasons for the discrepancy in priority with the client. Another aspect to take into consideration is that more than one nursing diagnosis can be addressed with a client at any given time. One diagnosis doe not have to be totally resolved before giving attention to another.

22. An observation nursing order is one that includes observations regarding potential complications as well as observations of the client's current status. A treatment nursing order is one that includes teaching, referrals, or physical care needed in the treatment of an existing problem.

Chapter 9

1. a

2. a

3. d, a, e, c, b

4. d

5. a

6. a

7. b

8. c

9. a

10. d

11. c

12. b

13. c

14. d

15. critical pathways, care maps

16. c

17. d

18. a

19. a. Home environment
    b. Client and family learning needs
    c. Need for skilled care
    d. Long-term care needs

20. d

© 2011 Cengage Learning. All Rights Reserved. May not be scanned, copied or duplicated, or posted to a publicly accessible website, in whole or in part.

Critical Thinking

21. The nurse needs three skills when implementing interventions. The first skill is cognitive. This skill is needed to make appropriate observations, understand the rationale for activities, and analyze how the differences between individuals influence nursing care. Critical thinking is an element of this skill. The second skill needed is psychomotor. This skill ensures that the nurse is able to physically perform the skills of client care such as administering medications and assisting with basic care and ambulation. The last skill the nurse needs is interpersonal. This skill is needed to communicate with clients and families as well as other health care professionals.

22. The nursing management system that would best support this design of client care unit would probably be team nursing. Team nursing uses a variety of personnel, with the registered nurse serving as the team leader, supervising team members, and planning and evaluating care activities. The registered nurse provides care to clients who are more acutely ill, while less skilled care providers care for more stable clients. Nursing assistants can provide basic care and perform other tasks as assigned by the team leader. This nursing management system would be the most cost-effective for this size and type of client care area.

Chapter 10

1. b, d, e	6. a, b	12. d
2. b	7. c	13. b
3. d	8. d	14. c
4. a	9. d	15. b
5. a	10. c	16. constructive, destructive
	11. b	17. d

Critical Thinking

18. The nurse who communicates with clients in a positive way will encourage open and honest communication when evaluating the success or lack of success of an intervention. The nurse who is negative or defensive will encourage clients to tell the nurse only what they believe the nurse wants to hear. This will lead to negative encounters and unsuccessful evaluations.

19. The evaluation process begins with establishing standards. These are specific criteria used to determine if a goal has been achieved. Next, data are collected. Assessment skills are needed to collect data that are focused on the goals and expected outcomes. Once the data are collected, the material needs to be analyzed to determine if the goal was achieved. This part of the process is validated by analyzing the client's responses to specific nursing interventions in the plan of care. Then, nursing actions are examined to determine their relevance to the client's needs and nursing diagnoses. With the use of critical thinking skills, the nursing interventions to improve the client's status are analyzed. The client's status is then reassessed and compared to the baseline data collected in the initial assessment. Finally, if necessary, the plan of care is modified.

© 2011 Cengage Learning. All Rights Reserved. May not be scanned, copied or duplicated, or posted to a publicly accessible website, in whole or in part.

Chapter 11

1. b

2. a. Certification of practice area
   b. Approved education programs such as BLS and ACLS

3. d

4. d, e, g, b, f, a, c

5. d

6. c

7. b

8. a

9. d

10. a

11. a. Licensure examination
    b. Continuing education
    c. Certification

12. c

13. d, c, a, b

14. b

15. b

16. b

17. b

18. b

19. c

20. b, c, e

Critical Thinking

21. The American Nurses Association's purpose is to improve the quality of nursing. This organization has activities to reach each area of nursing: practice, education, and research. The ANA establishes standards for nursing practice. It also develops educational standards and provides continuing education programs. The ANA promotes nursing research and has a professional code of ethics. In order for a nurse to become a member of the ANA, the nurse first needs to join his or her state nursing association. Regardless of the individual's area of interest, a nurse will find something in this organization to support it. The ANA also has a voice in legislation regarding health care and actively works to protect the economic and general welfare of registered nurses.

22. The politics of nursing does not mean that which occurs at the different branches of the government but rather refers to how things are done within an organization. Politics is the way in which people try to influence decision making, who controls the resources, and who is rewarded. Nurses can become more active in organizational politics by participating in committees, learning the unwritten rules of conduct, earning the appropriate credentials, becoming an effective communicator, networking, becoming active in a professional organization, and projecting a positive image of the profession.

Chapter 12

1. b

2. c, b, d, a, e

3. 2, 4, 1, 3

4. b

5. c

6. a

7. a

8. a

9. a

10. c

11. d

12. a. Failure to monitor client states
    b. Medication errors
    c. Falls
    d. Use of restraints

13. a

14. b

15. c

16. b

17. b

© 2011 Cengage Learning. All Rights Reserved. May not be scanned, copied or duplicated, or posted to a publicly accessible website, in whole or in part.

18. a

19. b

20. b

21. e, a, b, d, c

22. b

23. b

24. b, d, e, f, c, a

25. d

26. Informed consent, Refusal of treatment, Use of scarce resources, Impact of cost-containment initiatives, or Incompetent health care providers

27. d

28. d

29. b

30. a

31. c

32. d, a, b, c

33. a

34. a, b

35. a

36. a

Critical Thinking

37. An expert witness is a person called by the parties in a malpractice suit, is a member of the same profession as the party being sued, and is qualified to testify about the expected behaviors performed by members of the profession in a similar situation. The expert witness, in this situation, is a personal friend of the nurse being sued. The expert witness nurse has an obligation to the profession and society and therefore should serve as the expert witness in the case. The nurse being sued should understand the role of the expert witness and support the expert witness nurse's need to participate.

38. Understaffing is addressed by the Joint Commission standards, and the organization has guidelines that must be followed regarding safe client care. The nurse in charge should contact the nursing supervisor and discuss the issue regarding the temporary reduction in staffing for the shift. The nursing supervisor will need to obtain additional staff to cover the 4-hour deficit in staffing. The unit should not remain understaffed while the nurse is accompanying a client off of the unit.

Chapter 13

1. d

2. c

3. b

4. d

5. b

6. c

7. a

8. d

9. d

10. d

11. c

12. d, a, f, e, c, b

13. a

14. d

15. c

16. b

17. b

18. a

19. b

20. c

© 2011 Cengage Learning. All Rights Reserved. May not be scanned, copied or duplicated, or posted to a publicly accessible website, in whole or in part.

Critical Thinking

21. The use of computers has expanded over the last decade to include documentation, research, access to Web sites with instructional information, communication, and data management. The nurse today has to be familiar with computer terminology and at ease with the use of the equipment. Computers are now used during basic nursing education courses, so many nurses are prepared to use this technology once they have graduated. The nurse who may have not used computers during the basic nursing education might have difficulty transitioning to the use of computer technology when providing client care.

22. Telehealth is the use of telecommunication technology to provide client care. This technology includes computers, telephones, and monitoring devices. One might think that the purchase of the equipment would increase the cost of providing client care, but in the long run, the use of the technology will reduce the cost of client care. Clients can be monitored at home, which could prevent emergency room visits, hospitalizations, or prescribing practitioner office visits. Signs and symptoms can be reported faster, and interventions can be implemented sooner.

Chapter 14

1. a, b, c, e
2. a
3. b
4. Social, Therapeutic, Social, Social, Therapeutic
5. d
6. a
7. b
8. c
9. b, a, d, c
10. a
11. presence
12. b
13. d
14. c, b, a
15. b
16. d
17. c
18. a
19. a
20. d

Critical Thinking

21. Watson's theory of human caring is founded on the concept that caring is central to nursing practice. Emphasis is placed on the dignity and worth of individuals, and each person's response to illness is unique. Additional concepts in Watson's theory include the ideas that caring is demonstrated interpersonally, involves a commitment to care, and is based on knowledge. Benner's theory is founded on the concept that caring is central to all helping professions. According to Benner, caring is the foundation of being. Both Benner and Watson believe that all people's individual concerns are important. Benner believes that caring is communicated through actions, that problem solving is a major component of caring, and that advocacy is a form of caring.

22. A therapeutic relationship has the characteristics of warmth, hope, rapport, trust, empathy, acceptance, active listening, humor, compassion, self-awareness, a nonjudgmental approach, flexibility, and the ability to take risks. All of these characteristics are interpersonal relationship skills that the nurse needs to cultivate in order to establish a therapeutic relationship.

© 2011 Cengage Learning. All Rights Reserved. May not be scanned, copied or duplicated, or posted to a publicly accessible website, in whole or in part.

23. Active listening is listening that focuses on the speaker and is the basic skill for interpersonal effectiveness. Active listening is facilitated by attending behaviors—nonverbal skills that convey interest in what the other person is saying. The person who actively listens utilizes all three elements of communication: verbal, paraverbal, and nonverbal. Active listening focuses on the feelings behind the words and not just the words.

Chapter 15

1. b
2. b, a, e, d, c
3. b, c, a
4. d
5. d
6. d
7. a
8. d
9. b, d, c, a
10. a
11. e, c, f, b, d, a
12. c
13. c
14. a
15. d
16. d
17. d
18. c
19. c
20. a
21. b
22. c
23. d
24. a
25. He can hear what is being said to him.

Critical Thinking

26. Group dynamics is the study of events that take place during group interactions. These dynamics occur when nurses interact with families, treatment teams, therapy groups, committees, and coworkers. Group dynamics include nonverbal messages, seating, and interactions between the individuals within the group.

27. Touch is a powerful nonverbal method of communication that should be used cautiously with clients who are confused, aggressive, suspicious, or victims of abuse. A confused client may misinterpret the intent of the touch. An aggressive client may see the touch as a threat and lash out. A suspicious client may think the touch is harmful. And the victim of abuse may be frightened by touch.

Chapter 16

1. a, f, d, e, b, c
2. a
3. b
4. Treating the client as a unique individual,
5. 2, 4, 3, 1
   Protecting privacy and confidentiality, Using touch and personal space in a therapeutic manner, Respecting cultural differences, or Decreasing anxiety through stress management techniques
6. b, e, d, h, g, f, c, a
7. d
8. b
9. d
10. a

© 2011 Cengage Learning. All Rights Reserved. May not be scanned, copied or duplicated, or posted to a publicly accessible website, in whole or in part.

11. b, c, a, d	14. b	17. b
12. c	15. a	18. d
13. d	16. a	

Critical Thinking

19.   The clinical model of health is a traditional model that views health as an absence of illness. An individual who is not experiencing a disease or illness is considered healthy. In the health promotion model of health, there are activities that promote or improve wellness and prevent disability. Individuals use health-promoting activities when they value health, perceive health as being within their control, can identify benefits in self-care activities, and have a positive perception of their own health status.

20.   Becoming more responsible for one's own health means entering into a partnership with a health care provider to work together to achieve health status goals. In the past, individuals who were ill would seek the care of a health professional in order to "fix" the problem or illness. This philosophy of health care is changing. More people are changing previous unhealthy behaviors to those that support health.

Chapter 17	7. c	14. c
1. a, d, b, c	8. c	15. c
2. a	9. d	16. a
3. b	10. c	17. aggregate
4. a	11. a	18. c, c, b, a
5. a	12. d	19. a
6. dysfunctional	13. c	20. a

Critical Thinking

21.   The nurse should document the findings and report them to the appropriate protective services agencies. Documentation should include verbatim statements of the victim, photographs, and description of the injuries. The client should be provided with telephone numbers of local shelters and crisis hotlines. In addition, the client should be referred to mental health professionals for counseling. The nurse should conduct the assessment so that the victim feels safe in order to establish rapport and trust.

22.   A tornado is considered a natural disaster and greatly affects the community. The community health nurse should help determine the safety of all community members. Then, those with immediate medical needs should be addressed. From there, the nurse can assist with identifying how basic needs, such as food, water, and temporary housing, can be met. The community health nurse is aware that every community member is not going to receive the optimal services that he or she would in a different situation; however, the intention is to provide services for the greater good at this time.

© 2011 Cengage Learning. All Rights Reserved. May not be scanned, copied or duplicated, or posted to a publicly accessible website, in whole or in part.

Chapter 18

1. b
2. c
3. a
4. a
5. d
6. b, e, d, c, a
7. a, c, d
8. bond
9. d
10. c
11. 6, 7, 2, 3, 1, 5, 4
12. a
13. a
14. d
15. b
16. b
17. b
18. d
19. a
20. b
21. a

Critical Thinking

22. The CDC has identified a health protection goal for the five developmental stages. For infants and toddlers, the goal is to start strong. For children, the goal is to grow safe and strong. The adolescent goal is to achieve healthy independence. The adult goal is to live a healthy, productive, and satisfying life. And the goal for older adults and seniors is to live better, longer.

23. Adult clients can be subdivided into three age ranges. For those ages 19 to 49, the recommended immunizations are possibly a dose of tetanus, diphtheria, and pertussis; three doses of the human papillomavirus, if indicated, for females; one or two doses of measles, mumps, and rubella; an annual influenza vaccination; one or two doses of pneumococcal vaccine; doses of hepatitis A and hepatitis B; and one or more doses of meningococcal vaccine. The recommended vaccinations for adults from age 50 to 64 are the same as for those aged 19 to 49 except that the human papillomavirus vaccination is not indicated. For the last adult group, ages greater than 65 years, one dose of measles, mumps, and rubella; one dose of pneumococcal; doses of hepatitis A and B; one or more doses of meningococcal; and one dose of zoster are recommended.

Chapter 19

1. agism
2. d
3. e
4. a
5. a
6. d, a, c, b
7. a
8. d
9. a
10. a
11. d
12. c
13. b
14. a
15. c
16. b, c, d, g, f, a, e
17. d
18. a
19. Decreased visual acuity, Poor vision in dimly lit areas, Less foot and toe lift when walking, Altered center of gravity, Slower reflexes, Impaired muscle control, Orthostatic hypotension, or Urinary frequency
20. b

© 2011 Cengage Learning. All Rights Reserved. May not be scanned, copied or duplicated, or posted to a publicly accessible website, in whole or in part.

Critical Thinking

21. Because the elderly typically have more health problems that require medication for treatment, there is a risk of the elderly client not adhering to the prescribed medication regime. Ways to enhance an elderly client's adherence to medications include scheduling the medication to be taken around certain daily living activities to serve as a reminder to the client. Another way is to make sure the medications are accessible. The client can also prepare the medications a week in advance and store them in medication boxes, according to the day, to increase adherence. In addition, the client can talk with the pharmacy to see if the medications can be dispensed in packets or groupings so that the client will know that one packet will be taken each day.

22. The elderly client is a victim of exploitation, which is a dishonest or inappropriate use of an older person's money. This is a form of abuse. What makes this situation worse is that the client is giving her money to a son in lieu of purchasing required medications. The nurse needs to intervene and report this situation to Adult Protective Services. The nurse also should contact Social Services to see if there are any elderly medication assistance programs that the client might be eligible for to assist with obtaining the needed medications.

Chapter 20

1. a, f, d, e, c, b
2. b
3. communication
4. d, c, a, b
5. b
6. d
7. c
8. d
9. c
10. b
11. b
12. d, a, e, c, b
13. a
14. c
15. d
16. a
17. d
18. b
19. c

Critical Thinking

20. Ethnocentrism is the belief that one's culture is superior to all others. When this occurs, it can lead to oppression. Oppression is when the rules, modes, and ideals of one group are imposed on another group. Oppression can lead to racism, which is discrimination directed toward individuals who are misperceived to be inferior due to biologic differences. When ethnocentrism occurs, those who are not viewed as superior are treated as being less valued than those in the culture believed to be superior. This will lead to disrespect and lack of regard for those not of the culture believed to be superior.

21. In people of the African, Asian, or Native American cultures, isoniazid—a drug used to treat tuberculosis—is rapidly metabolized. This causes the drug to become inactive very quickly, which means it will not remain in the body long enough to treat the disease. Additional medication treatment or dose adjustments will need to be made for individuals within these cultural groups who are diagnosed with tuberculosis.

© 2011 Cengage Learning. All Rights Reserved. May not be scanned, copied or duplicated, or posted to a publicly accessible website, in whole or in part.

Chapter 21

1. d

2. b

3. d

4. b

5. d

6. kinesthetic

7. a, c, d, b

8. c

9. c

10. a

11. b

12. d

13. d

14. d

15. c

16. a

17. b

18. d

19. learning plateau

20. c

Critical Thinking

21. There are four major categories of client education. The first is health promotion. This category covers the topics of parenting skills, nutrition, exercise, and family planning. In the category of health restoration, topics include medication information, community resources, and information about treatment modalities. For the next category, illness and injury prevention, topics range from immunizations, health screening, smoking cessation, and breast self-examination to safety measures. The final category is facilitating coping. In this category, topics such as the safe use of medical equipment, dietary modifications, information about disease processes, counseling, and stress management are included.

22. Repetition is one of the principles of learning and is needed to retain material. Repetition reinforces practice. Repetition also means providing or presenting the same material in a variety of ways to ensure that the client has learned the information.

Chapter 22

1. d, a, b, c

2. d

3. d

4. c

5. d

6. b

7. b

8. c

9. b

10. d

11. b

12. a

13. a

14. a

15. a

16. d

17. c

Critical Thinking

18. The role of the nurse is that of caregiver. Because the nurse is constantly putting the needs of clients first, this behavior can easily be transferred into the nurse's personal life. The major indication that a nurse is developing personal low self-esteem is that he or she denies or minimizes his or her own needs and puts the needs of another first. In addition, the profession of nursing has been combating the

© 2011 Cengage Learning. All Rights Reserved. May not be scanned, copied or duplicated, or posted to a publicly accessible website, in whole or in part.

negativity associated with being a "handmaiden" to the profession of medicine. A nurse who is already prone to having personal low self-esteem is at risk for developing feelings of worthlessness if confronted by an aggressive prescribing practitioner.

19. The nurse needs to make clear statements of expected behavior by explaining procedures and telling the client what to expect and what will occur. Additional ways to support a client's self-esteem include respecting privacy, treating each client as an individual of worth, and encouraging the client to maintain as much independence as possible while the nurse provides assistance as needed.

Chapter 23

1. a, c, g, d, h, e, f, b
2. c
3. b
4. a
5. a
6. b
7. d
8. c
9. f, a, e, g, d, h, c, b
10. secondary gain
11. d
12. b
13. a
14. b
15. a
16. a, c, b
17. d
18. d
19. a
20. b

Critical Thinking

21. With mild anxiety, the person has an increased degree of alertness and increased vigilance. This is an optimal time for that person because he or she is more aware and has an increase in the perceptual fields. In severe anxiety, the person has selective attention and distorted perception. The person experiencing severe anxiety has difficulty remembering information and is prone to making less than optimal decisions or plans.

22. There are several reasons why a person resists change. The first reason is conformity or going along with others to avoid conflict. The next is because of dissimilar beliefs and values, which are different for each individual. Fear of the unknown is another reason why people resist change. Habits, or a routine set of behaviors, are the most difficult to change. Another reason is satisfaction with the status quo. With this reasoning, the person cannot see how the change will make things better when conditions are fine the way they are. Secondary gains are another reason to resist change. In this rationale, the person gets special benefits or rewards for the current conditions and cannot see the benefits of changing. Change might lead to threats to the satisfaction of basic needs. And last, a person might resist change because the change represents unrealistic goals or sets the person up for failure.

Chapter 24

1. A relationship with a higher power, oneself, and significant others
2. d
3. d
4. c
5. a
6. b, a, b, a, b, a
7. d

© 2011 Cengage Learning. All Rights Reserved. May not be scanned, copied or duplicated, or posted to a publicly accessible website, in whole or in part.

8. trust

9. a state experienced when an individual perceives that his or her belief system, or place in it, is threatened.

10. a, b, c

11. c

12. a

13. b, a, c, d

14. b, a, c

15. d

16. Self-alienation, Loneliness/social alienation, Anxiety, Sociocultural deprivation, Pain, Death, Life changes, Chronic illness

17. d

18. Mindfulness

19. b

20. a

21. a. *Spiritual distress*
    b. *Risk for spiritual distress*
    c. *Readiness for enhanced spiritual well-being*

Critical Thinking

22. The nurse needs to approach the care of this client the same as for every other client, by being nonjudgmental and encouraging a trusting relationship to establish rapport. The client's statement does not reflect what he "does" believe in, so the nurse could ask the client to explain what he does to support his spiritual needs. The nurse can do this by utilizing the spiritual assessment tool that assesses the dimensions of meaning and purpose, inner strengths, and interconnectedness.

23. Faith is a belief in and a relationship with a higher power and is demonstrated by either spirituality or religiosity. Hope is a factor that enables one to cope with distressing events. Faith and hope are interconnected. Faith is expecting that what one hopes for will be realized. Hope is a characteristic of faith. Both exist together.

Chapter 25

1. g, f, a, b, e, d, c

2. b, c

3. a

4. a

5. b

6. a

7. d

8. b

9. a

10. b

11. d, e, c, b, a

12. b

13. a

14. a

15. a

16. b, a, c

17. c

18. c

19. b

20. c

Critical Thinking

21. Lindemann's theory of grief has five stages. The first stage is somatic distress. In this stage, the person experiences episodic waves of discomfort that last from 10 to 60 minutes. The person also experiences somatic complaints and emotional pain. The second stage is that of preoccupation with the image of the deceased. The person has a sense of unreality, demonstrates an emotional detachment from others, and

© 2011 Cengage Learning. All Rights Reserved. May not be scanned, copied or duplicated, or posted to a publicly accessible website, in whole or in part.

has an overwhelming preoccupation of visualizing the deceased. The third stage is guilt. In this stage, the bereaved considers the death to be a result of his or her own negligence or lack of attentiveness. There is also an active search for evidence of how he or she could have contributed to the death. The fourth stage includes hostile reactions. In this stage, relationships with others become impaired, which causes the bereaved to be left alone. The last stage is loss of patterns of conduct. In this stage, the bereaved is unable to sit still and continually searches for something to do.

22. In an unexpected or unanticipated death, there is no closure. The survivors are shocked and bereaved and did not have the chance to say "good-bye." In a traumatic death, such as in the case of a suicide, the survivors suffer emotions of greater intensity. There may be traumatic imagery, which is reliving the terror of the incident or imagining the feelings of horror felt by the victim. Traumatic imagery can lead to posttraumatic stress disorder. Unless the problem is identified and addressed, the person will not be able to progress through the normal grieving process.

Chapter 26

1. c

2. c, a, f, d, e, g, b

3. c

4. b

5. d

6. a

7. d

8. a

9. a

10. a

11. b, d, a, f, c, g, e, h

12. b

13. c

14. c

15. a

16. d

17. 80

18. d

19. c

20. a

Critical Thinking

21. This is a stage 1 hypertension reading that needs to be validated. First, permit the client to sit quietly for several minutes before reassessing the blood pressure. This will give the client's body time to adjust to the change in posture from ambulating to sitting. The nurse should ensure that the correct size of blood pressure cuff is used. The nurse should also review the technique to ensure that the bladder of the cuff is appropriately placed. Once all of this has been done, the nurse should reassess the client's blood pressure. Then, the nurse should assess the blood pressure using the client's other arm to determine which reading to use. A diagnosis of hypertension cannot be made on one blood pressure reading.

22. Because of damage caused to the hypothalamus from central nervous system trauma, bleeding, or increased intracranial pressure, a client with a traumatic brain injury can develop neurogenic fever. This is a long-term elevation of the body temperature believed to be caused by an interruption in the body's normal temperature set point. The nurse should frequently monitor the temperature of a client with a brain injury to facilitate early diagnosis and early treatment if temperature elevation is present.

© 2011 Cengage Learning. All Rights Reserved. May not be scanned, copied or duplicated, or posted to a publicly accessible website, in whole or in part.

Chapter 27

1. d
2. 2, 3, 4, 1
3. c
4. a
5. c, e, b, d, a
6. b
7. a
8. d
9. b
10. d
11. a
12. cystocele
13. d
14. Fat, Fluid, Flatus, Feces, Fetus, Fatal growth, Fibroid tumor
15. d
16. d, a, b, c
17. stereognosis
18. c
19. c
20. a

Critical Thinking

21. The general survey includes the observation of any acute problem such as difficulty breathing, holding a body part, sweating, pallor or cyanosis, or the appearance of being anxious. The client's general state of health, stature, and sexual development should be observed. From there, the nurse should assess the client's height, weight, and vital signs. The general survey also includes the client's posture, motor activity, gait, manner of dress, hygiene, personal grooming, and detection of any body or breath odors. The client's facial expressions and behaviors should be observed along with the client's manner, affect, and reaction to persons and/or things in the environment. Last, the nurse should assess the client's quality of speech and level of consciousness.

22. The nurse uses the senses of sight, touch, hearing, and smell when gathering information during the physical assessment. Sight is used to observe the client's body, behaviors, movement, and motor dexterity. The sense of touch is used when performing palpation. The back of the hand is used for assessing temperature. The skin pads of the fingers are used to palpate the size, position, and consistency of various body parts. Touch is also used when conducting percussion. Hearing is used when performing auscultation and listening to what the clients say about their health status. The nurse uses the sense of smell to assess any body or fluid odors.

Chapter 28

1. b
2. a
3. b
4. c
5. c
6. d
7. c
8. a
9. a
10. c
11. a
12. a
13. d
14. b
15. c
16. d
17. a
18. b
19. c
20. c, d, g, f, e, h, b, i, a, j
21. b, c

© 2011 Cengage Learning. All Rights Reserved. May not be scanned, copied or duplicated, or posted to a publicly accessible website, in whole or in part.

Critical Thinking

22. LDL is the major cholesterol carrier in the blood. When too much LDL circulates in the blood, it can slowly build up in the walls of the arteries and cause the formation of atherosclerotic plaques, which can clog the arteries. This type of cholesterol is often referred to as "bad" cholesterol. HDL accounts for approximately one-fourth of the body's cholesterol and carries the cholesterol away from the arteries and back to the liver, where it is removed from the blood. HDL removes excess cholesterol from atherosclerotic plaques and slows their growth. HDL is often referred to as "good" cholesterol because the higher the value, the lower the incidence of coronary heart disease.

23. Client teaching before a diagnostic test should include the reason for the test, what to expect, an estimated length of time the test will take, whether the client needs to take nothing by mouth before or during the test, if the client needs to take a bowel preparation prior to the test, how to generate sputum if needed for the test, if a urine specimen will be needed, whether to arrive at the test without any jewelry or hair clips, if a contrast medium will be used and how it will taste if taken orally, if a contrast medium will be injected and how it will feel to the client, positioning during the test, positioning after the test, and if fluids can be taken after the test is completed.

Chapter 29

1. f, a, e, g, h, d, c, b

2. c, b, a, d, e

3. a

4. b

5. b

6. b

7. a

8. d

9. handwashing with antimicrobial soap, alcohol-based hand rub

10. b

11. a

12. b

13. d

14. 10, 7, 9, 1, 3, 4, 8, 6, 5, 2

15. c

16. a. To protect the client
    b. To allow for treatment in a safe environment
    c. To reduce the risk of injury to others

17. d

18. c

19. b, c, a

20. c

Critical Thinking

21. Being in the hospital can produce anxiety; however, anxiety can become worse when a client is in isolation. The nurse needs to address the client's psychological needs by explaining the isolation precautions and rationales. The nurse should also discuss the client's feelings about being isolated. While communicating with the client, the nurse needs to convey empathy and understanding. To help reduce the client's feelings of loneliness, the nurse should visit with the client and permit visitors to visit as long as isolation precautions are followed. The nurse should also assess and support whatever the client needs to help reduce the feelings of loneliness.

© 2011 Cengage Learning. All Rights Reserved. May not be scanned, copied or duplicated, or posted to a publicly accessible website, in whole or in part.

22. This act, which went into effect in October 2008, states that Medicare will no longer reimburse hospitals at a higher rate for the increased costs that result from hospital-acquired conditions (HACs). Medicare will, however, pay for prescribing practitioners and other covered items or services that are needed to treat the HACs, including postacute care. Hospitals will lose money if a client develops an HAC. Medicare and Medicaid believe that HACs are really "never events" or, rather, events that should never occur in a hospital. Many of these events can be avoided by following good safety practices, infection control, and basic client care such as turning, repositioning, early postoperative ambulation, and frequent assessment of client health status.

Chapter 30

1. d
2. c
3. a
4. Distribution
5. c, b, a, d
6. b
7. c
8. c
9. c
10. d
11. d
12. b
13. b
14. a
15. a. Right drug
    b. Right dose
    c. Right client
    d. Right route
    e. Right time
16. b
17. c
18. c
19. c
20. a
21. c
22. a
23. d
24. a
25. c

Critical Thinking

26. The right documentation means that the nurse correctly documents that the medication was provided to the client. The documentation could be on the medication administration record as well as within a nurses' note. If written in a nurses' note, the documentation might include the client's need for the medication (such as a request for pain medication) and the client's response to the medication after receiving it (such as pain reduced, on a scale of 1 to 10, from an 8 to a 3 after receiving the medication).

27. A nurse who is drug impaired may demonstrate suspicious behavior such as insisting on carrying the narcotic keys and volunteering to administer all of the narcotics for a group of clients during a shift. Other behaviors include exhibiting extreme and rapid mood swings, always wearing long sleeves, signing out more controlled drugs than anyone else, reporting frequent spills and breaking of controlled drugs, committing multiple medication errors, practicing illogical or sloppy charting, frequent absence from work, coming to work early and staying late, and frequently using sick days.

© 2011 Cengage Learning. All Rights Reserved. May not be scanned, copied or duplicated, or posted to a publicly accessible website, in whole or in part.

Chapter 31

1. b
2. b
3. b
4. a
5. c
6. Imagery
7. a
8. b
9. 5, 3, 2, 1, 4
10. a
11. a
12. a
13. c
14. a
15. d
16. b
17. d
18. d
19. c
20. aromatherapy

Critical Thinking

21. Although the use of alternative therapies is growing, many are not accepted by mainstream medical practitioners. The client has found an alternative therapy that is assisting him with managing the pain associated with headaches and wishes not to share this information with his prescribing practitioner for fear of reprisal or criticism. The nurse should support this client's decision but should encourage the client to discuss this healing therapy with the prescribing practitioner to maintain open communication and ongoing support to meet health goals.

22. Reflexology is based on the fundamental belief that the foot is a microcosm of the entire body. In reflexology, illness is manifested by calcium deposits and other acids that are deposited in the corresponding part of the person's foot. Massaging the foot or pressing on areas of the foot stimulates energy movement by relieving accumulated toxins in the corresponding body part. The inserts that the client is using could be stimulating corresponding body parts, causing the client to feel relaxed.

Chapter 32

1. c
2. d
3. d
4. SaO_2
5. b
6. b
7. c
8. b
9. b
10. d
11. a
12. atelectasis
13. c
14. c
15. d
16. a
17. huffing
18. d
19. b
20. c

Critical Thinking

21. An endotracheal tube has to be inflated to sit securely within a client's trachea. If a client is agitated, there is a risk that the client will accidentally remove the endotracheal tube, causing traumatic injury and occlusion of the airway. The client who is agitated might need to be restrained either physically or

© 2011 Cengage Learning. All Rights Reserved. May not be scanned, copied or duplicated, or posted to a publicly accessible website, in whole or in part.

chemically. Chemical restraint is a type of sedation in which the client will not be agitated. Physical restraint is the application of wrist restraints to the client to prevent the movement of the hands to the location of the endotracheal tube. The use of restraints must be accomplished according to organizational policies and in adherence to the policies of the Joint Commission and other regulatory bodies.

22. The presence of oxygen increases the risk of fire because it is a catalyst for fire to occur. The presence of any fuel along with a source of ignition, such as a spark from a lighter or a lit cigarette, will lead to fire more rapidly. The client should be instructed to ask his wife not to smoke in the presence of oxygen equipment.

Chapter 33

1. d, a, b, c
2. b
3. b
4. b
5. a, c
6. a
7. b
8. a
9. a
10. a
11. a
12. c
13. c
14. d
15. a
16. a
17. b
18. b
19. b
20. b
21. a
22. c
23. a
24. d
25. a
26. b
27. d
28. b
29. b
30. c, d, a, b

Critical Thinking

31. The body has three main control systems to regulate acid-base balance: the buffer systems, respiratory regulation, and renal regulation. Several chemical buffer systems of body fluids are activated under different conditions. The bicarbonate-carbonic acid system is the primary buffer system. In this system, the body responds to a change in acid-base balance by increasing either carbonic acid or bicarbonate. Respiratory regulation helps to maintain acid-base balance by controlling the content of carbon dioxide in extracellular fluid. This is done by either increasing or decreasing respirations. The kidneys control extracellular fluid pH by eliminating either hydrogen ions or bicarbonate ions from body fluids.

32. Several elements of the health history are necessary to assess a client's fluid balance. These elements are lifestyle; dietary intake; religion; weight; fluid output; gastrointestinal disturbances; fever; diaphoresis; presence of draining wounds, burns, or trauma; disease conditions that could upset the fluid balance; and therapeutic programs that could upset the balance.

© 2011 Cengage Learning. All Rights Reserved. May not be scanned, copied or duplicated, or posted to a publicly accessible website, in whole or in part.

Chapter 34

1. a
2. d
3. d
4. a
5. d
6. e, h, a, g, f, b, c, d
7. a
8. a
9. b
10. c
11. a
12. c
13. 3, 2, 1, 4
14. b
15. d
16. d
17. c
18. b
19. b
20. c
21. a
22. a, c, e, d, f, g, b
23. a
24. d, c, b, a
25. a. Biological
    b. Psychological
    c. Economic

Critical Thinking

26. The jejunum is approximately 4 feet in length. The nutrients that are absorbed in this region of the gastrointestinal tract include riboflavin, thiamin, vitamin C, and monosaccharides. The client who has had several feet of the jejunum removed because of disease will not have the maximum amount of these nutrients absorbed from foods eaten and will need to have supplementation to maintain adequate levels in the body. Of these nutrients, the one that will have the greatest impact on health is vitamin C, which could affect the blood, healing, and normal functioning of the musculoskeletal and neurological systems.

27. Refeeding syndrome is a complication that can occur during the initial phase of enteral nutrition, of parenteral nutrition, with oral intake, or from dextrose-containing intravenous fluids. It occurs primarily in severely malnourished clients due to electrolyte and fluid imbalances because the body is not used to having the correct amounts of nutrients. When nutritional therapy is started and nutrients are provided, the body responds with shifts of electrolytes and fluid. The electrolytes for which this syndrome is most often seen include phosphorous, magnesium, and potassium. The client can develop cardiac complications and, after a few days or weeks, neurological complications. To avoid refeeding syndrome, efforts at improving a client's nutritional status should be done slowly.

Chapter 35

1. subjective
2. a
3. b
4. d
5. b
6. d
7. c
8. a
9. b
10. d
11. a, e, b, d, c
12. c
13. a
14. c
15. b, c, a
16. a
17. b
18. e, a, b, f, d, c
19. b
20. a

© 2011 Cengage Learning. All Rights Reserved. May not be scanned, copied or duplicated, or posted to a publicly accessible website, in whole or in part.

Critical Thinking

21. There are two states of sleep: non–rapid eye movement and rapid eye movement. Non–rapid eye movement sleep has four stages. In stage 1, sleep is light and lasts approximately 10 minutes. Stage 2 is also fairly light sleep. Fifty percent of all sleep is in this stage. The next two stages, 3 and 4, occur almost simultaneously. Stage 3 is medium-depth sleep, and stage 4 is the deepest sleep. If a person is aroused during this stage of sleep, he or she may take up to 15 seconds to become fully awake. Stages 3 and 4 of sleep are the most restorative sleep and are needed for physical recovery. Rapid eye movement sleep occurs after approximately 90 minutes of sleeping. The heart and respiratory rates are irregular and often higher than when awake, even though the body is immobilized. Dreams occur during 80% of the time the person is in this sleep state. This period of sleep becomes longer as the night progresses and the person becomes more rested. It occurs during approximately 20% to 25% of all time spent in sleep.

22. Pharmacological agents that might be helpful for a client with a sleep disturbance include tricyclic antidepressants, antihistamines, and short-acting hypnotics. Tricyclic antidepressants improve a client's ability to fall asleep and stay asleep by causing sedation when given 1 to 3 hours before bedtime. Antihistamines have mild sedative effects that could promote sleep if given at bedtime. Short-acting hypnotics promote sleep and should be prescribed only on a short-term basis.

Chapter 36

1. b
2. c
3. b
4. a
5. d
6. c, d, f, e, b, a
7. absorption of nutrients and excretion of wastes
8. d
9. a
10. c
11. d
12. d
13. a contracture
14. c
15. 2 hours
16. c
17. b
18. c
19. c
20. b

Critical Thinking

21. With exercise, the heart becomes more efficient as it adapts to increased demands for oxygen, and the cardiac output increases. In addition, there is a decrease in resting heart rate and resting blood pressure. Immobility increases the workload on the heart, increasing heart rate and blood pressure. Lack of exercise can lead to thrombi formation due to blood pooling in the extremities and can cause orthostatic hypotension, or a drop in blood pressure when a person changes position. This is because of decreased vessel tone.

22. The three concepts that nurses need to be aware of when positioning clients are pressure, friction, and skin shear. A pressure site is any skin surface on which a client is lying or sitting. The force of the pressure can reduce circulation and lead to skin breakdown and ulceration. Friction is caused when the skin is dragged across a rough surface. Friction causes heat, which can damage the skin and lead to decreased skin integrity. Skin shear is the result of dragging skin across a hard surface. The force of resistance tears the deep layers of skin, which can lead to skin ulceration.

© 2011 Cengage Learning. All Rights Reserved. May not be scanned, copied or duplicated, or posted to a publicly accessible website, in whole or in part.

Chapter 37

1. b

2. d, f, a, b, e, c

3. b

4. wound healing

5. c

6. a

7. c

8. b

9. a

10. a

11. c

12. c

13. a. *Anxiety*
    b. *Deficient knowledge*
    c. *Body image disturbance*

14. d

15. c

16. c

17. d

18. b

19. e

20. b

Critical Thinking

21. Pressure ulcers are staged so that the degree of tissue damage can be classified. There are four stages of pressure ulcers. Stage I is described as nonblanching redness of intact skin. This is the precursor to a pressure ulcer. Stage II is considered partial-thickness skin loss of the epidermis or dermis. The ulcer is superficial and appears like an abrasion, a blister, or a shallow crater. In stage III, there is full-thickness skin loss involving damage or necrosis of subcutaneous tissue that may extend to but not through the fascia. In stage IV, there is extensive destruction. The skin loss is full thickness with tissue necrosis and damage to the muscle, bone, or other supporting structures. Undermining and sinus tracts may also be seen in a stage IV pressure ulcer.

22. The Braden Scale for Predicting Pressure Sore Risk evaluates six criteria: sensory perception, moisture, activity, mobility, nutrition, and friction and shear. Each criterion is rated on a scale of 1 to 4. The lower the score, the greater the risk for pressure ulcer development. The Norton Scale for Pressure Ulcer Risk evaluates five criteria: physical condition, mental condition, activity, mobility, and incontinence. Each criterion is rated on a scale of 1 to 4, and the lower the score, the greater the risk for pressure ulcer development.

Chapter 38

1. c

2. b

3. d

4. c

5. b

6. a

7. a

8. b

9. d

10. c

11. a

12. b

13. a

14. b

15. c

16. d

17. b

18. a

19. b

20. d

© 2011 Cengage Learning. All Rights Reserved. May not be scanned, copied or duplicated, or posted to a publicly accessible website, in whole or in part.

Critical Thinking

21. The Glasgow Coma Scale is divided into the assessment of three behaviors. The first behavior is best eye-opening response. The client is scored according to the response as being spontaneous, to verbal command, to pain, or to no response. The second behavior is that of best verbal response. The client's response is scored as being oriented/conversing, being disoriented/conversing, using inappropriate words, making incomprehensible sounds, or having no response. The last behavior in the scale is best motor response. The client is scored as obeying verbal commands, moving to localized pain, demonstrating flexion withdrawal to pain, demonstrating abnormal posturing—decorticate, demonstrating abnormal posturing—decerebrate, or having no response. The higher the score a client receives, the greater the orientation to the environment.

22. There are four groups of herbs that benefit the nervous system. The first is tonics. Herbs in this category nourish, tone, and strengthen the nervous tissue and cells. They are also high in calcium, magnesium, the B vitamins, and protein. To be most effective, these herbs should be taken over a long period of time. The second category is nerve demulcents. These herbs soothe and heal irritated and inflamed nerve endings. The next category is nerve sedatives, which relax the nervous system by reducing pain and tension and promote sleep. The final category is nerve stimulants. Herbs in this category activate nerve endings by increasing circulation, providing nutrients, and revitalizing the nervous system.

Chapter 39

1. e, a, f, h, b, d, c, g

2. a

3. a

4. a

5. a

6. a

7. d

8. ability to maintain a tight seal

9. b

10. a

11. b

12. d

13. b

14. a

15. a

16. c

17. 2, 1, 2, 2, 1, 2, 1

18. notify the prescribing practitioner

19. b

20. c

Critical Thinking

21. As a person ages, muscle tone is lost. In addition, an older client is more likely to have functional limitations, such as impaired mobility, that can contribute to an alteration in bowel elimination. Elderly clients have a diminished perceived desire to defecate and a prolonged colonic transit time. Medications that this population might be prescribed—such as narcotics, sedatives, anticholinergics, antidepressants, and other medications to treat specific health problems—can contribute to the development of constipation. On the other hand, an elderly client might be treated with antibiotics for an acute infectious condition that could cause diarrhea. Also, an elderly client might be receiving enteral feedings, which are known to cause diarrhea because of their osmolality.

© 2011 Cengage Learning. All Rights Reserved. May not be scanned, copied or duplicated, or posted to a publicly accessible website, in whole or in part.

22. Intrinsic sphincter deficiency is a disorder of the muscular components of the urethral sphincter. With a radical prostatectomy, the innervation to the sphincter is interrupted, leading to total incontinence. Since this often cannot be avoided because of the surgery, the client should be instructed on what to expect regarding urine output, what can be done to help protect his skin and clothing, and products available that he can wear to collect or absorb the urine.

Chapter 40

1. a	9. a	18. c
2. d, e, c, b, a	10. b	19. d
3. c	11. a, c, b	20. a
4. c, a, d, b	12. c	21. d
5. a	13. c	22. a
6. d	14. embolus	23. b
7. c	15. c	24. b
8. b	16. b	25. d
	17. d, a, e, c, b	

Critical Thinking

26. The scrub nurse wears sterile attire; prepares the instrument tray; and passes the instruments, sponges, needles, and sutures to the surgeon. The circulating nurse wears clean attire and obtains supplies, delivers materials, pours solutions, handles specimens, positions the client and surgical drapes, disposes of soiled items, and coordinates the care of the client. Both nurses are responsible for counting the number of used instruments, needles, and sponges, which is to be done before the surgeon closes the incision. This is to ensure that nothing is accidentally left inside the operative site.

27. Each health care organization has its own criteria to determine when a client can be extubated after receiving general anesthesia; however, some general guidelines are followed. The client should be able to lift his or her head off of the bed for 5 seconds. The client should also be able to produce strong bilateral hand grasps. The nurse will measure the client's inspiration force and vital capacity. Oxygen saturation is also measured, in addition to the presence of bilateral breath sounds. Once these criteria have been met, the anesthesiologist explains the extubation procedure to the client and conducts the procedure.

© 2011 Cengage Learning. All Rights Reserved. May not be scanned, copied or duplicated, or posted to a publicly accessible website, in whole or in part.